Care of Drug Users in General Practice

A harm reduction approach

Second Edition

Edited by

Berry Beaumont
General Practitioner

Foreword by

David Haslam
Chairman of Council
Royal College of General Practitioners

Radcliffe Publishing
Oxford • San Francisco

Radcliffe Publishing Ltd
18 Marcham Road
Abingdon
Oxon OX14 1AA
United Kingdom

www.radcliffe-oxford.com
Electronic catalogue and worldwide online ordering.

British Library Cataloguing in Publication Data

A catalogue record for this book is available from the British Library.

ISBN 1 85775 624 X

Typeset by Action Publishing Technology Ltd, Gloucester
Printed and bound by TJ International Ltd, Padstow, Cornwall

Contents

Foreword

Drug abuse is a nightmare feature of the 21st century. From tabloid headlines to crime statistics, this is a problem that makes most of us feel a sense of genuine despair. Pessimism and hopelessness are often rife. Good news is all too rare.

But there is one area of hugely positive news relating to illegal drug abuse. The recent quite remarkable upsurge in interest by general practitioners and other members of the primary healthcare team in learning about how to tackle this problem is a huge counter to the prevailing pessimism. In the last few years over a thousand clinicians have been through the RCGP's Certificate in the Management of Drug Misuse training course and many more have expressed an interest in becoming involved. At a time of apparently low national morale in general practice, of a dreadful workforce crisis and countless and increasing demands on the team's time, it is even more remarkable that so many doctors, nurses and pharmacists have chosen to develop expertise in this vital area of care.

For primary care to become involved is completely appropriate. Few conditions exemplify more clearly the need for a generalist holistic approach to a problem. It has been estimated that some 50 000 drug users received treatment in a primary care setting in the year 2003 and, as Clare Gerada and Tom Waller write in their overview in this remarkable book, as a result of medical or other problems related to drug misuse, GPs may come in contact with users of a wide variety of drugs, often at a relatively early stage in their drug-taking career.

Whilst the natural inclination to shrug and say that this problem is too great for GPs to deal with is completely understandable, nevertheless general practitioners who have developed skills to manage problems related to drug use are in a unique position to facilitate change. Drug abusers may be the unhealthiest members of the population, with physical and mental health factors compounding their drug problems. Whether the problems are depression, infection, diet, hygiene, childhood abuse, unemployment or any one of the other ills that flesh is heir to, the person who abuses illegal drugs is likely to have more health-related problems than almost anyone else.

However, despite this obvious need there is a huge risk that this particular group of our population will suffer from the inevitable consequences of the inverse care law. This states that 'the availability of good medical care tends to vary inversely with the need for it in the population served'.[1] Or, as the Bible puts it: 'Unto every one that hath shall be given, and he shall have abundance; but from him that hath not shall be taken away even that which he hath'. Could there be a more cogent and convincing reason for high-quality GPs and high-quality primary care teams to get involved?

With most medical conditions, clinicians feel nervous and uneasy until their knowledge and skill base is adequate. Caring for road traffic accidents or emergencies in childbirth make most of us nervous, because we lack experience and exposure. But drug abuse is becoming such a major part of our society that involvement of practices is becoming more and more pressing.

The fact that this excellent book has reached its second edition is a measure of the interest that GPs and primary care teams are now showing in this topic and the speed with which knowledge and drug abuse, are changing. I commend it unreservedly.

David Haslam
Chairman of Council
Royal College of General Practitioners
April 2004

■ Reference

1 Hart JT (1971) The inverse care law. *Lancet.* **i**: 405–12.

List of contributors

Dima Abdulrahim
Specialist Adviser
National Treatment Agency
Hannibal House
Elephant and Castle
London SE1 6TE

Tom Aldridge
Young Person's Manager
National Treatment Agency
Hannibal House
Elephant and Castle
London SE1 6TE

Jean-Claude Barjolin
Primary Care Development Adviser
SMMGP (Substance Misuse Management in General Practice)
c/o Trafford Substance Misuse Services
1–3 Ashton Lane
Sale
Manchester M33 6WT

Jim Barnard
Primary Care Adviser
SMMGP (Substance Misuse Management in General Practice)
c/o Trafford Substance Misuse Services
1–3 Ashton Lane
Sale
Manchester M33 6WT

Dr Berry Beaumont
Non-executive Director
National Treatment Agency
General Practitioner
The Surgery
2 Mitchison Road
London N1 3NG

Dr Judy Bury
Primary Care Facilitator (HIV/Drugs)
Lothian Primary Care Trust
Spittal Street Centre
22–24 Spittal Street
Edinburgh EH3 9DU

Dr Tom Carnwath
Consultant Psychiatrist
County Durham Substance Misuse Service
Pierremont Unit
Hollyhurst Road
Darlington DL3 6HX

Kate Davies
Co-ordinator, Nottinghamshire County Drug and Alcohol Team
5a Beech House
Ramsom Wood Business Park
Southwell Road West
Rainworth
Mansfield NG21 0ER

Vivienne Evans
Chief Executive, Adfam
Waterbridge House
32–34 Loman Street
London SE1 0EH

Dr Chris Ford
General Practitioner
Chair RCGP Sex, Drugs and HIV Task Group
GP Adviser, SMMGP (Substance Misuse Management in General Practice)
Lonsdale Medical Centre
24 Lonsdale Road
London NW6 6RR

Dr Clare Gerada
Project Director
RCGP National Drug Misuse Training Programme
Frazer House
32–38 Leman Street
London E1 8EW

Dr Linda Harris
Clinical Director, Primary Care Substance Misuse
Wakefield Integrated Substance Misuse Services
Grosvenor House
Union Street
Wakefield WF1 3AE

Dr Mary Hepburn
Senior Lecturer in Women's Reproductive Health
Consultant Obstetrician and Gynaecologist
University of Glasgow
Princess Royal Maternity Hospital
Alexandra Parade
Glasgow G31 2ER

Alan Joyce
Senior Advocate, The Methadone Alliance
c/o The Alliance
PO Box 32168
London N4 1XP

Dr Jenny Keen
Clinical Director, Primary Care Clinic for Drug Dependence, Sheffield
Clinical Research Fellow, Institute of General Practice and Primary Care,
University of Sheffield
Guernsey House
84 Guernsey Road
Sheffield S2 4HG

Dr Katie Kemp
Specialist in Primary Care
Camden and Islington Substance Misuse Services
Primary Care Unit
St James's House
109 Hampstead Road
London NW1 2LS

Christina McArthur
Primary Care Adviser
SMMGP (Substance Misuse Management in General Practice)
c/o Trafford Substance Misuse Services
1–3 Ashton Lane
Sale
Manchester M33 6WT

Dr Gordon Morse
Medical Consultant to Clouds House
RCGP Regional Lead, South West England
Riversdale
High Street
Fovant
Salisbury
Wiltshire SP3 5JL

Greg Poulter
Director, DETRU
11 Doverfield Road
Guildford GU4 7YF

Jane Powell
Children's Guardian
Senior Development Officer, National Children's Bureau
PO Box 44605
London N16 6XD

Sue Tyhurst
Services Manager
Brighton Oasis Project
22 Richmond Place
Brighton BN2 9NA

Dr Tom Waller
Formerly, Suffolk County Specialist in Substance Use
Died 27.11.03

Brian Whitehead
Counsellor in General Practice
Lonsdale Medical Centre
24 Lonsdale Road
London NW6 6RR

Dr Nat Wright
GP Consultant in Substance Misuse
Centre for Research in Primary Care
71–75 Clarendon Road
Leeds LS2 9PL

Acknowledgements

I would like to thank everyone who has contributed to this book. The Substance Misuse Training Programme of the Royal College of General Practitioners has provided generous financial support. Thanks must also go to the drug-using patients in my practice who have trusted me to provide their care. I have learnt a lot from listening to them. I hope everyone who reads this book will do the same.

Dr Berry Beaumont
April 2004

CHAPTER 1

A GP's role: past, present and future

Clare Gerada and Tom Waller

■ Introduction

National policy for the care of drug users in general practice has undergone considerable change in recent years and is continuing to evolve. In the space of 25 years the treatment of opiate dependency by primary care practitioners has moved from indifference, with few able or willing to get involved, to a position where primary care leads the way, with an estimated 50 000 drug users receiving treatment in a primary care setting in the year 2003.

As a result of medical or other problems related to drug misuse, GPs may come in contact with users of a wide variety of drugs, often at a relatively early stage in their drug-taking career. GPs who have developed skills to manage problems related to drug use are in a good position to facilitate change. Of paramount importance is a constructive doctor–patient relationship. General practitioners do not need to know every small detail of every drug of misuse. This book will demystify and give insights on how to manage users of different groups of drugs but drug problems are essentially people problems and the knowledge and skills that GPs have developed to help their patients with other problems will be of most help. Substitute prescribing, if it is needed, is an easily learnt technique and is usually best done on a shared-care basis with the local drug service, which will act as a source of expert advice and support. Treating drug users can be a heavy burden on time but with realistic expectations, reducing harm to both the individual and the local community through small, progressive goals makes it well worthwhile. Working in a general practice setting to help a patient minimise the harm from drug dependence, earning the deep-felt gratitude of the person concerned, their family and close friends can be a very rewarding experience.

■ Setting the scene: harm reduction

As drug taking becomes more common, so the likelihood increases that medical, social, psychological or legal problems will develop. The harm caused by these problems affects not only individual drug users but also their family and friends and the community within which they live, whether or not they are acquainted with the drug taker concerned.

It is now widely recognised that the harm associated with these problems can be reduced by appropriate professional input and that this is a much more constructive approach than treatments that aim at chemical abstinence alone. The way forward needs to be on a broad front, with appropriate co-ordinated professional input into the social, psychological, criminal and medical aspects of drug taking. This is best done as a partnership approach, not only for the treatment of individual drug users but also on a locality basis by local organisations and through the work of drug action teams. Some of the health harm to individual drug users can be reduced by GPs providing general medical services and further harm reduction can be achieved either by working together with or by referral to specialist drug services.

Nevertheless, many GPs have concerns over their roles when drug users attend surgery asking for help. What is the most appropriate help for them to provide and where do their responsibilities end under general medical services? These concerns are addressed throughout this book and are at first best viewed in the context of developments that have taken place in UK national policy.

■ Historical developments

In 1912, Britain signed the Hague Convention and in doing so gave an international commitment to control the supply of certain narcotic and other drugs. The first defined legislation on drugs of dependence in the UK, the Dangerous Drugs Act, followed in 1920. This Act allowed doctors to use narcotic drugs for *bona fide* medical treatment but unfortunately did not state whether this included the treatment of drug dependence. A Departmental Committee on Morphine and Heroin Addicts was set up to sort out this issue and was chaired by Sir Humphrey Rolleston, the then President of the Royal College of Physicians. The Departmental Committee's deliberations were published in 1926 and became known as the Rolleston Report.[1] This was the first defined policy on the treatment of drug dependence in the UK. It was a flexible policy and was envied by physicians in many other countries, such as the USA, where a doctor's clinical freedom to treat opiate addicts in the way he or she felt was most appropriate was curtailed by restrictive legislation. The Rolleston Report outlined the following two indications for the use of morphine or heroin in the treatment of drug dependence.

- If the person was being gradually withdrawn.
- If, after attempts at cure had failed, the patient could lead a normal and useful life when provided with a regular supply but ceased to do so when the supply was withdrawn.

Thus the principle of maintenance treatment was born and this became known as 'the British system'. The number of opiate addicts in the UK at that time was relatively small. Before the 1950s there were so few heroin addicts in Britain that nearly all of them were known personally to the Home Office Drugs Branch Inspectorate, which periodically checked pharmacy records. There were several exaggerated press reports about the danger to the British public of Chinese opium dens in London's docklands but in reality almost all opiate dependence in the UK was probably due to prolonged prescribing of morphine by doctors. From 1926 until the late 1950s, the number of people who were being helped to lead normal and useful lives through the British system (usually on an injectable diamorphine prescription) was stable, varying between 400 and 600. These people were mainly middle class and middle aged or elderly.

■ The Brain Committee reports

Around 1960, reports began to emerge of a new group of opiate drug takers. These were young people, mainly in their late teens and 20s, who were misusing and advocating the use of prescribed drugs for 'kicks'. An Interdepartmental Committee on Drug Addiction chaired by Sir Russell Brain was set up to look into this matter and reported in 1961 that the drug situation in Britain gave little cause for concern.[2] However, media coverage continued and the committee was asked to reconvene. In 1965, the second Brain Committee reported very differently that a new, young, unstable, non-therapeutic group of drug takers had emerged and that although some illicitly produced drugs were sold on the street, much of the problem was caused through overprescribing of therapeutic drugs by unscrupulous, uninformed or vulnerable doctors open to blackmail. The second Brain Committee[3] recommended that where possible, prescribing should be taken out of the hands of GPs and instead carried out by specialist psychiatrists, who would work from special centres to be known as drug dependence units (DDUs).

The DDUs were set up between1968 and 1970 in densely populated inner-city areas, mainly in London. They were few in number and almost exclusively confined to England. Only one specialist centre for drug users was established in Wales and none at all in Scotland and Northern Ireland. Since not all areas of the country could be covered by the new specialist psychiatrists, general psychiatrists and GPs, although discouraged, were not completely prevented from treating drug users.

By the late 1970s the number of drug users, far from falling, had shown a rapid rise. There were several reasons for this.

- Cheap and plentiful supplies of illicitly produced heroin from abundant harvests in Pakistan and the Far East.
- The appeal of high-gain, low-risk operations enticed criminal gangs (who had previously avoided this area of activity) to start drug trafficking.
- The widespread introduction of the new habit of smoking heroin ('chasing the dragon') as opposed to injecting or sniffing it.

The rapid increase in numbers of opiate users seeking help caused the specialist services to become overwhelmed. The British system of maintenance prescribing was questioned and by the early 1980s, the specialist clinics almost all moved over to rigid detoxification regimes of a maximum duration of 3–6 months.

Almost four decades since the introduction of DDUs, the relentless increase in illicit drug use has continued, particularly among young people, in spite of many efforts to contain it. Every year the situation has worsened, in the UK and throughout the world, and the prevalence of drug use has shown a consistent inexorable increase, year on year. During this time many changes have taken place in the UK treatment services.

■ The impact of HIV

The fear of an AIDS epidemic in the late 1980s brought about a change in policy in relation to the treatment of drug users. A working party of the Advisory Committee on the Misuse of Drugs (ACMD) was set up in 1987 to report on the issues in relation to HIV and AIDS and to make recommendations. The first of three reports on acquired immune deficiency syndrome (AIDS) and drug misuse was published in 1988.[4] It was highly influential and led to a major change in the way that drug services worked with patients. The report stated a fundamental principle that it was more important to both the individual and the public health to limit the spread of HIV within the drug-using population than to overcome the drug problem itself. Harm reduction was to take precedence over abstinence and although abstinence was not forgotten, there was a hierarchy of other goals that were more important to achieve. An example of this hierarchy for individual drug users might be:

1 the cessation of sharing injecting equipment
2 the cessation of injecting
3 reduction of drug use
4 abstinence.

It was now seen as vital to be proactive rather than reactive, so that services could reach as many drug users as possible, including those who did not wish to stop using drugs, to help them reduce the risk of contracting and spreading HIV disease both through shared injecting practices and sexually. It was recommended that outreach services and facilities for the promotion of needle exchange were introduced. General practitioners were seen as a key resource because of their widespread accessibility and because they would be one of the first ports of call when drug problems began to develop. They were thus in a good position to reduce the spread of HIV at an early stage, both by giving harm reduction advice and by prescribing oral opiate substitute drugs, such as methadone mixture, to opiate injectors.

One of the recommendations was to give more back-up resources to GPs by the provision of community drug teams (CDTs) in every health district who would work with GPs on a shared-care basis. The CDTs would perform a counselling and non-prescribing function and the GP would look after the medical side of the treatment package. The teams would be a source of expert advice for GPs, if required, and would work closely with GPs on individual cases. This package of measures is now recognised as having been highly successful in helping to limit the epidemic of HIV in drug users and reducing its spread into the general hetero-sexual population.[5] There is, however, no room for complacency as a much larger epidemic of hepatitis C has surfaced. Six out of every 10 users with a history of injecting who attend UK drug services are hepatitis C positive.[6] These figures cover not just opiate users who inject but also injectors of a wide range of other drugs including amphetamine, cocaine and benzodiazepines.

■ National policy and general practitioners' management of drug misuse

■ Targets

Over the years, policy makers have been attempting to get general practitioners more involved in the care of drug users.[7,8] The government's drugs strategy[9] calls for at least 30% of GPs to be involved in the care of this patient group. Surveys of GP involvement do show an upward trend, from 5% in 1986[10] to 23% in 2003[11] willing to provide substitute medication to drug users. However, numbers are still not at the levels demanded by national targets.[12]

■ Roles and responsibilities

With regard to the GP's role, the current approach is best summarised in the recommendations of the 1996 Task Force Report,[8] the National Clinical Guidelines[13] and the National Treatment Agency's *Models of Care*.[14] The recommendations contained in these documents are broadly those listed below.

- GPs have responsibility for the physical health needs of drug users within the provision of general medical services and should be encouraged to identify drug misuse, promote harm reduction and, where appropriate, refer to specialist services.
- The process of shared care, with appropriate support for GPs, should be available as widely as possible. Primary care trusts (PCTs) (and their forerunners health authorities) should encourage its expansion to enable GPs to take overall clinical responsibility for drug users and agree with a specialist a treatment plan that may involve the GP prescribing substitute opiate drugs.
- GPs should be sufficiently skilled to identify problem drug users who may be consulting them for other, perhaps related, problems. This may require a programme of training for some GPs.
- GPs should know to whom they can refer drug users in a crisis and for ongoing support, either from specialist drug workers regularly attending their clinics or by access to a named key worker in the local specialist agency.
- The service provided by the GP should be agreed with the Local Medical Committee (LMC) and specialist services and should clearly set out the respective roles of the GP and the specialist services and the support the GP can expect in delivering the service. GPs should have straightforward access to urine-testing facilities.
- Where they have concerns about the patient taking or storing the prescribed medication appropriately, GPs should have access to facilities where supervised consumption can take place.
- The agreement for the provision of shared care made between the LMC and local drug providers, such as specialists and general practitioners with special clinical interest, should include arrangements for referral, assessment and management. Primary care trusts should monitor local arrangements and ensure adequate controls are in place.

- Where the service is defined as a Nationally Enhanced Service (www.bma.org.uk), additional payments should be provided as agreed with the PCT and LMC.

■ Standards

The National Clinical Guidelines for the treatment of drug misuse and dependence include a number of recommendations aimed at improving safety through:

- good assessment procedures
- urine testing
- daily dispensing
- supervised ingestion.

In 2000, the ACMD published its report *Reducing Drug Related Deaths*,[15] which recommended an attitudinal shift in thinking amongst the drug treatment agencies to one of embracing cessation of injecting as its core policy. For primary care, the recommendations centre on improving prescribing practice and reducing diversion of prescribed drugs.

■ Levels of service provision

The clinical guidelines assumed that GPs would work within the context of shared care and categorised practitioners into three levels of expertise: the generalist, the specialist-generalist and the specialist. Definitions of these levels of service provision are contained within the guidelines but basically they involve an increasing level of expertise and clinical care. *The NHS Plan*[16] emphasises the need to create new roles for practitioners, in particular general practitioners with a special clinical interest (GPwSI), doctors who are able to support others and provide 'enhanced' services. These GPwSIs can be seen as congruent with the specialist-generalist of the Drug Misuse Clinical Guidelines.[17]

■ Non-governmental drivers
■ Policy statements

At a Royal College of General Practitioners' conference on managing drug users in general practice in 1996, the following consensus statement was agreed.

- All GPs should offer GMS to drug users.
- All GPs should be willing to assess drug misuse problems and refer patients as appropriate.
- Where GPs take on an extended role in the care of drug users, this should be resourced in recognition of the extra workload involved.
- There is an urgent need for training about drug misuse to be included in 'core medical training' at an undergraduate level. There is also a need for

continuing medical education in this area for all GP registrars, GPs and hospital doctors.

The Royal College of General Practitioners / General Practitioner Committee policy statement on the care of substance users was published in April 2000. This proved to be a watershed with the profession publicly acknowledging that they have a role in the care of drug users. The statement highlights the need to accept drug users into treatment, albeit with the support of shared care, training and additional resources.

RCGP/GPC requirements for GP involvement

- GPs have had additional training in such treatment.
- GPs are supported by a specialist team for updates and supervision.
- The service is funded from outside the GMS pool.
- Supervised consumption facilities are available.

■ Training

Through a grant obtained from the Department of Health (England), the Royal College of General Practitioners has developed, delivered and accredited a Certificate in the Management of Drug Misuse aimed at general practitioners with special clinical interest in drug misuse. This is the first accredited post-graduate qualification from the RCGP. The Certificate is an eight-day training programme, delivered over 4–6 months, using a variety of teaching methods (including didactic lecture-based training and small group master classes led by experienced GPs). To date, nearly 1000 GPs and other professionals have passed through the training programme. The RCGP is now developing a foundation course, to be called Part 1 of the Certificate, aimed at equipping generalist practitioners with the necessary skills and knowledge to deliver services competently at a generalist level.

■ The changing role of the GP

The new general medical service (GMS) contract[18] has defined a primary care service for drug users as a nationally enhanced service. This is a service which can be commissioned by the PCT from local practices with national minimum specifications and benchmark pricing. PCTs are not required to commission this service if local circumstances and/or financial constraints suggest there are other priorities, nor would all practices within a PCT be required to provide it if it was commissioned. At the time of writing the details of the nationally enhanced service and how they translate into practice still need to be worked out. It is our belief that the new contract has mixed blessings. On the one hand, drug users can now expect to receive high-quality care from practitioners contracted to provide enhanced services; on the other hand, the bounty attached to the head of each drug user in treatment is unlikely to be met by every health organisation who, faced with financial constraints, will be forced for the first time to ration primary care drug misuse services.

The new contract recognises a long-held view that GPs should receive additional payment for seeing and treating drug users, provided they adhere to minimum standards of care and have undertaken appropriate training. The implementation of this new contract could encourage many more GPs from all over the country to participate in additional training in the treatment of problem drug use. In addition, locally agreed protocols and guidelines should assist GPs in providing high-quality professional treatment of drug users. It is to be hoped, but is by no means certain, that increasing numbers of GPs will become involved in caring for drug users. A potential workforce of around 40 000 GPs would make a significant impact on the problem.

Key points

- Primary care is aptly suited to the care of drug users.
- Primary care practitioners need training, support and resources to do this work well.
- The new GMS contract and the development of general practitioners with special clinical interest give new opportunities for the primary care workforce to get involved.
- Primary care's involvement in the next decade should be not 'whether' but 'how?'

■ Acknowledgement

Tom Waller died on 27.11.2003. He was a pioneer in the harm reduction movement and was providing care to drug users in general practice long before it was common practice. He was the driving force in setting up 'Action on Hepatitis C'. In 2001 the UK Harm Reduction Alliance established an annual award in his name. He will be sadly missed.

■ References

1 Spear B (1994) The early years of the 'British System' in practice. In: J Strang and M Gossop (eds) *Heroin Addiction and Drug Policy. The British system*. Oxford University Press, Oxford.
2 UK Interdepartmental Committee on Drug Addiction (1961) *Report*. (Chaired by Sir Russell Brain.) HMSO, London.
3 UK Interdepartmental Committee on Drug Addiction (1965) *Second Report*. (Chaired by Sir Russell Brain.) HMSO, London.
4 Advisory Council on the Misuse of Drugs (1988) *AIDS and Drug Misuse Part 1*. HMSO, London.
5 Stimson GV (1996) Has the United Kingdom averted an epidemic of HIV-1 infection among drug injectors? *Addiction* **91** (8): 1085–8.
6 Judd A, Hickman M, Renton A *et al.* (1999) Hepatitis C virus infection among injecting drug users: has harm minimisation worked? *Addiction Research*. **7**: 1–6.

7 Advisory Council on the Misuse of Drugs (1993) *Aids and Drug Misuse – update*. HMSO, London.

8 Task Force to Review Services for Drug Users (1966) *Report of an Independent Review of Drug Treatment Services in England*. Department of Health, London.

9 Department of Health (1998) *Tackling Drugs to Build a Better Britain: the Government's ten-year strategy for tackling drug misuse*. Stationery Office, London.

10 Glanz A and Friendship C (1990) *The Role of GPs in the Treatment of Drug Misuse. Findings from a survey of GPs in England and Wales*. Report prepared for the Department of Health, London.

11 National Treatment Agency (2003) *Analysis of Drug Action Team Treatment Plan Returns*. NTA, London. Available online at: www.nta.nhs.uk

12 Audit Commission (2002) *Changing Habits. The commissioning and management of community drug treatment services for adults*. Audit Commission, London. Available online at: www.audit-commission.gov.uk

13 Department of Health, Scottish Office Department of Health, Welsh Office, Department of Health and Social Services, Northern Ireland (1999) *Drug Misuse and Dependence – guidelines on clinical management*. Stationery Office, London. Available online at: www.drugs.gov.uk/polguide.htm

14 National Treatment Agency (2002) *Models of Care for Treatment of Adult Drug Users*. NTA, London. Available online at: www.nta.nhs.uk

15 Home Office (2000) *Reducing Drug Related Deaths – a report by the Advisory Council on the Misuse of Drugs*. Stationery Office, London.

16 Department of Health (2000) *The NHS Plan. A plan for investment, a plan for reform*. Stationery Office, London. Available online at: www.doh.gov.uk/nhsplan/index.htm

17 Gerada C, Wright N and Keen J (2002) The general practitioner with a special clinical interest: new opportunities or the end of the general practitioner? *Br J Gen Pract*. **52**: 796–7.

18 British Medical Association, NHS Confederation (2003) *Investing in General Practice: the new General Medical Services Contract*. BMA/NHS Confederation, London. Available online at: www.bma.org

CHAPTER 2

Assessment of the drug user

Chris Ford and Brian Whitehead

A good-quality assessment is the basis for providing appropriate care to drug users and their families in general practice. GPs and primary healthcare teams are increasingly likely to be consulted by drug users and are a first point of contact for many.[1] General practice is in a unique position to provide services to whole families and GPs are ideally located to respond to a wide variety of their needs. GPs see a broader and more varied range of drug users than many of the specialist treatment services that have traditionally focused on long-term opiate users. Primary care has the capacity to deal with a range of presenting problems and is experienced in the management of chronic relapsing conditions. GPs have many transferable skills already learnt in the management of other chronic conditions such as diabetes and asthma. The uniqueness of primary care is the potential length of time we have to support and treat drug users and their families. We work in a distinctive environment that cares for people from the cradle to the grave and is second to none in assessing and managing risk.

Assessment is the mutual gathering of information to assess the patient's needs and to assist in defining the most appropriate course of action. It is an ongoing process rather than a one-off event, as the individual's needs evolve over time. Decisions about the treatment of individual patients and determining the most appropriate interventions should be based on a thorough assessment of what will work for that person and on reliable information on what works generally. The assessment does not all have to be done at once but timely intervention is essential to effect optimal outcome. 'Effective assessment needs to be tailored in terms of comprehensiveness and complexity in such a way that it does not present a barrier to entry to, and engagement in, appropriate drug and alcohol treatment.'[2]

Benefits of a comprehensive assessment

- Allows a profile of the patient and their drug problem to be developed.
- Helps the drug user to think about:
  - why they are using drugs
  - why they are presenting now
  - what they may need to change.
- Helps identify the patient's health and social needs.

Continued overleaf

- Helps identify the most appropriate treatment plan for the indi
- Helps identify treatment goals.
- Helps decide whether this patient can/should be treated in practice. This will be informed by:
  - the experience of the GP
  - relationships with local services
  - the ability to refer to additional services.

■ Levels of involvement

The primary care team needs to consider what level of involvement with drug users is appropriate for their practice. They also need to consider the extent of their competence and ability before they become involved in certain aspects of the treatment of drug users, such as substitute prescribing.

Possible levels of GP involvement[3]

1 No provision of services to illicit drug users.
2 Provision of GMS only.
3 Provision of drug-related interventions under direct supervision.
4 Provision of drug-related interventions with specialist support as required.
5 The GP with a special interest.

Taking on the care of a long-term dependent heroin drug user, a crack user in crisis or a polydrug user is a totally different proposition from providing advice to a recreational weekend ecstasy user. There are likely to be a number of problems of a physical, psychological and social nature in those drug users who have been dependent on illicit drugs for longer periods.

Accept your limits and define your philosophy/boundaries

Match your patients

What can I do? What can't I do?
What will I do? What won't I do?
With what do I need help? Where can I get it?

- Are you able to commit to an increased workload and consultation time?
- Are you prepared to work long term with drug users, perhaps over many years, to effect change?
- Are you clear and comfortable with the philosophy of treatment/care that influences your interventions?
- Are you aware of the evidence base?
- Are you clear about your aims (abstinence or maintenance)?
- Are these compatible with the needs of your patients?

■ Factors to consider before deciding to treat a drug user in general practice

- *Knowledge of the patient*: do you know the patient and/or family? Has the patient self presented or been referred to you for treatment?
- *Type of drug use*: is drug use experimental, recreational, problematic or dependent? Not all drug use requires prescribing and prescribing is not all you can offer.
- *Length of drug use*: is drug use short, medium or long term? Shorter term drug use may be more manageable. However, with experience and support, long-term drug users can be managed in general practice.[4]
- *How many drugs*: using which drugs? Use of only one drug does occur but is increasingly infrequent.
- *Amount of drugs*: what is the level of drug use for each drug and is it manageable?
- *Social*: what social support do they have – partner, family and friends? Non-using partner or friends?
- *Housing*: does the person have suitable and secure housing?
- *Criminal*: is the person in a cycle of crime to fund their habit?
- *Health status*: is health compromised by their drug use? Consider medical conditions, e.g. HIV/hepatitis C.
- *Dual diagnosis/co-morbidity*: does the person have any confirmed mental illness?
- *Address*: does the person live in the practice area?

Patients who may need referral to specialist agencies

- Need high degree of intervention and/or counselling.
- Need help with other problems: housing, benefits.
- Have concurrent mental illness.
- Other addictions, e.g. alcohol.
- Using a combination of different drugs.
- If you do not feel experienced enough to initiate treatment.

■ Assessment in the GP surgery

A full assessment can be done by the GP over several consultations to fit in with normal surgeries or undertaken by a shared-care drugs worker or other appropriate person. Harm reduction information, such as advice on safer injecting, needle exchanges and immunisation, can be offered from the first meeting.

At assessment the GP needs to be able to:

- establish that the patient is using drugs and the type of drug use – experimental, recreational, problematic or dependent
- identify what drugs, what route? Why using? (Assess the amounts being taken and degree of dependence)
- offer brief interventions that provide specific advice on risk and harm reduction
- identify what problems and concerns are present
- assess the patient's motivation in relation to these problems and concerns
- determine if the patient's drug use is causing health or social problems.

It is now known that the sooner appropriate treatment begins, the better the outcomes. The assessment, especially with drugs like crack, can be seen as part of the treatment plan. However, it is important not to be forced into substitute prescribing before you have undertaken the necessary assessment and feel ready to begin treatment. Patients have often been managing their drug problem for some time and it is better to take the necessary time to assess and formulate a treatment plan.

Necessary checks before starting treatment

- An explanation to the drug user about why these checks need to be undertaken.
- The name and address of the patient.
- Proof of residency to be provided.
- The urine screen result to arrive (this may be impractical in areas where results take a long time – instant multi-stick screens should be used instead).
- The drug user to be sure if treatment is wanted.
- The GP to decide if this user can be managed in general practice.

■ The assessment process

- The drug and medical history.
- Examination.
- Screening for drug use.
- Other investigations.
- Notification.

The drug and medical history (see also 1999 clinical guidelines[5])

Why has the patient presented to you now?
- Why has the patient come to you?
- Why now? Is there a health, social or legal problem?

- Have friends, family, probation sent them or are they coming for themselves?
- What do they want (it may not always be drugs)?
- What do they see as the problem?
- How is their substance use impacting on their life?
- What do you see as the problem?
- Are you willing to help with the drug problem?
- Are you willing to help with any other health and social problems?

How has the patient presented?
- Outside surgery hours?
- With an arranged appointment?
- With a friend who is registered?
- As an emergency/in crisis?
- As a temporary resident?
- In obvious withdrawal?

Assessment of their current drug use (last four weeks)
- What drugs have they taken in the past month?
- What is their primary drug, how much and how often are they taking it?
- What other drugs and alcohol are they using, how much and how often?
- How are they taking the drugs (route of use: oral, smoking, chasing, snorting, skin popping, intravenous)?
- Are any drugs being currently prescribed?

Past drug history
- At what age did the user start taking drugs (including alcohol, cannabis and nicotine)?
- When did drug taking become a problem?
- What was the progression from one type of drug to another?
- What combination of drugs has been used?
- What are the reasons for taking one drug over another?
- What do drugs do for them?
- Has the drug user ever been abstinent from their drug of choice? When and for how long?
- If yes, how was this possible?
- What level of control do they have over their use?

Previous treatments
- Have they had previous treatment?
- What, when and for how long?
- Has treatment been as inpatient, rehabilitation, specialist service or primary care?
- Did they achieve abstinence and for how long?
- Do they know why they relapsed?
- What worked/didn't work for them?
- Have they had any contact with other services such as needle exchanges or street agencies?
- Why are they returning for treatment now?

Assessing risk-taking behaviour

- Do they ever inject? Are they injecting safely?
- Have they shared/lent needles, syringes or other paraphernalia, such as spoons or filters? Regularly, occasionally, frequently? NB: Don't forget to go into detail here because sometimes sharing with a partner is not seen as sharing.
- Where do they obtain their equipment: needle exchange, pharmacy?
- If they are reusing equipment, what are their current cleaning techniques?
- Are they currently in a sexual relationship: regular, casual or both?
- What is the sex of partner/s?
- Do they practise safer or unsafe sex?
- Do they use condoms and where do they obtain them?
- Are they aware of HIV, hepatitis B and C and how these viruses are transmitted?
- Have they ever been immunised against hepatitis A or B?

Assessment of physical health

- Do they have any medical problems: acute, chronic?
- Have they suffered any complications of their drug use such as abscesses, thrombosis, septicaemia, fits, chest or heart problems, hepatitis?
- Do they know their hepatitis A, B and C and HIV status?
- Are they on any prescribed medication?
- When did they last have a BP, peak flow rate, smear and contraception check?

Assessment of psychological health and motivation

- What are their primary concerns?
- What do they recognise as the problem?
- What do they want to change (current problem)?
- What do they want from change?
- Are they ready for change?
- Can they do it?
- What are their strategies for change?
- What are their strategies for coping?

Assessment of mental health

- Are they depressed or psychotic?
- Do they have any history of psychiatric disorder or have they had any contact with psychiatric services recently or in the past?
- Have they any history of overdoses – accidental or deliberate?

Assessment of social situation

- Personal relationships, partner, family, friends, children?
- Using/non-using partner, using/non-using friends?
- Contact with family?
- Any substance use in partner or other family member?
- Do they have children: how many, ages, where and with whom do they live?
- Accommodation: secure/homeless?
- What type of accommodation: private rented, council, housing association, owned, squat?

- Are there problems with the housing: crowded, damp, unsuitable?
- What is their level of schooling and qualifications?
- Employment history: what/how long? Any casual work? Hopes for employment?
- What is their financial situation?
- What is their income – benefits/work/debts?

Assessment of forensic history
- Have they had any contact, past or present, with the criminal justice system?
- Are there any outstanding charges?
- Have they ever been in prison and if so, when and for how long?
- Are they on probation?
- How is drug habit financed (remember confidentiality and explain)?

Goal setting

- Important to identify goals so that treatment has direction and focus.
- Goals need to be identified collaboratively with the patient so that both parties are clear about what is to be achieved.
- Goals should be specific, attainable and measurable and can be split into short and long term.
- Goals should start with the areas of risk: reducing illicit drug use, reducing levels of injecting and sharing.
- Help patient to think about how these changes may be brought about.
- Assessment is a process and should be sequential and ongoing as an individual's needs evolve over time.
- At the beginning, set a review date within the week and then review at regular intervals.

Physical examination
See Chapter 3.

Urine screening
A urine drug screen is an essential safeguard and helpful tool that should always be obtained at the outset of treatment and randomly through the course of treatment. For a laboratory analysis, 50 ml of urine is required and results take between seven and 21 days to return. Multi-sticks are increasingly available in general practice and can give a result in a couple of minutes. Both methods confirm drug use and should be done along with the history and examination. False negatives and false positives can occur, especially with the multi-sticks, so results should always be confirmed and interpreted in light of the history and examination.

Why do urine screens?
- To confirm that patient is using drugs and which ones.
- To help decide on the treatment plan.
- For your medicolegal protection.

- For the patient's protection.
- To help reduce street diversion.
- To encourage honesty; repeat if very different from the patient's story. False results do occur.

When asked, a group of users in Glasgow said they valued having their urine tested because it showed someone cared enough to bother to check their story (personal communication, Glasgow Drug Users Group, 1996). Many studies show greater than 94% concordance between history and urine results when the results are not used punitively.

What does urine testing tell us?
- The range of drugs being used.
- Not how much of a drug is being used. It is a qualitative result not a quantitative measure (some laboratories can measure quantities if specifically requested).
- If the user is dependent; opiates persist in urine up to 24 hours, methadone up to 48 hours, cocaine 24–48 hours (Table 2.1). If urine is negative and there is no clinical evidence of withdrawing, the user is not dependent.

When to do urine screens
- When a drug user presents (even if you are not going to prescribe), as a useful baseline or for future comparison.
- To confirm use before starting a substitute prescription.
- Before restarting a script after a break in treatment or relapse.
- At random throughout treatment to check on actual drug use against stated use.

Table 2.1 Drugs and their approximate detection times in urine

Drug	Detection time
Heroin/Morphine (Heroin is detected as a morphine metabolite)	1–3 days (possibly only one day)
Methadone (low dose)	1–2 days
Methadone (maintenance dose)	7–9 days
Dihydrocodeine	2–3 days
Codeine	2–3 days
Amphetamines	1–2 days (can be detected up to 4 days)
Methamphetamine	1–2 days
Cocaine/crack	12 hours–3 days
Benzodiazepines	
• Short acting (temazepam, chlordiazepoxide)	40–80 hours
• Long acting (diazepam, nitrazepam)	5–7 days
Barbiturates	Days–weeks (depending on type)
Cannabis	
• Casual use 1–4x/week	3–4 days
• Daily use	10 days
• Chronic heavy use	21–27 days
Ecstasy	2–4 days
Buprenorphine (not currently available from all laboratories)	2–3 days
Alcohol	12–24 hours

Factors affecting the time drugs can be detected in the urine
• The drug.
• The amount of drug taken.
• Single dose or chronic use.
• Other drugs taken.
• Taken with alcohol (enzyme inducer, metabolises and removes the prime drug faster).
• The concentration of urine (the reason why a creatinine is done at the same time).

Some specialist services have their own screening facilities. It may be possible to make an arrangement to use them.

Other available tests
• *Hair testing*: can give information covering drug use over weeks or months.
• *Mouth swabs*: increasingly available and less invasive.

Other investigations
See Chapter 3.

Notification
All patients presenting with a drug problem should be reported to the National Drug Treatment Monitoring System (NDTMS). The NDTMS came under the control of the National Treatment Agency in 2003 in England. Reporting is voluntary but underreporting could jeopardise the amount of funding made available to local services, which is partly allocated on the basis of the number of people in treatment.

The form consists of two copies; the top copy is for your records, the second copy should be sent to the local database (address on the form). Notification will become electronic in the future.

Confidentiality should be assured because the NDTMS copy does not include name or address. Nevertheless, it is good practice to explain to the patient what you are doing and why, and obtain consent.

Key points

• A good-quality assessment is the basis for providing appropriate care to drug users (and their family) in general practice.
• It is the mutual gathering of information to assess the patient's needs and to assist in defining the most appropriate course of action.
• Assessment is an ongoing process rather than a one-off event, as the individual's needs evolve over time.
• It includes taking an adequate history, conducting a brief examination for confirmatory evidence and carrying out a urine drug analysis.

■ References

1 Stimson GV, Hayden D, Hunter G *et al.* (1996) Drug users' help-seeking and views of services. In: Task Force to Review Services for Drug Misusers. *Report of an Independent Review of Drug Treatment Services in England.* Department of Health, London.

2 National Treatment Agency (2002) *Models of Care for Treatment of Adult Drug Users.* NTA, London. Available online at www.nta.nhs.uk

3 Resource and Service Development Centre (1995) *Shared Care, Shared Barriers. Reviewing shared care arrangements for drug misusers.* RSDC, Leeds.

4 Bury J (1995) Supporting GPs in Lothian to care for drug users. *Int J Drug Policy.* **6**(4): 267–73.

5 Department of Health, Scottish Office Department of Health, Welsh Office, Department of Health and Social Services, Northern Ireland (1999) *Drug Misuse and Dependence – guidelines on clinical management.* Stationery Office, London. Available online at: www.drugs.gov.uk/polguide.htm

CHAPTER 3

General healthcare of drug users

Katie Kemp

Substance misuse remains a growing problem and each year notifications to regional databases continue to rise.[1] Although urban areas have the highest prevalence of drug users, rural GPs are also likely to encounter ill health related to illicit drug use in their patients. Few would disagree that we have an important role in providing general medical care to drug users, whether or not the GP feels able to treat the drug dependency itself. Drug users registered with a general practitioner who is also treating their drug dependency consult their doctor more frequently than non-drug using patients.[2,3] This places GPs in a key position to detect and treat ill health in substance misusers and provides opportunities to screen for infectious and transmissible disease, immunise against preventable diseases such as hepatitis A and B and educate about the risks associated with illicit drug use. This chapter will focus predominantly on the physical ill health that may result from the use of Class A drugs such as heroin and cocaine but it should not be forgotten that many drug users undertake poly-drug use and that both alcohol and tobacco are also important contributors to illness in this patient group.

Morbidity and mortality are greatly increased in those misusing drugs, especially those injecting drugs and practising unsafe sex.[4] Accepting substance misusers onto their lists may significantly increase demands upon GPs' time and medical skills. The illnesses to which many such people succumb include all forms of viral hepatitis, bacterial endocarditis, HIV, tuberculosis, septicaemia, pneumonia, deep venous thrombosis, pulmonary emboli and abscesses, to name but a few. The difficulty for the GP is that many of the serious infections that may commonly occur in intravenous drug users are now uncommon in the rest of the population. This may hinder our ability to recognise illnesses which we rarely see and have little experience of treating. Despite the difficulties and increased workload involved, GPs report positively on their experience of providing treatment to drug misusers.[5,6]

■ Assessing the physical health of the substance misuser

It is helpful to make a full assessment of the substance misuser's general health as early as possible after acceptance onto the list. Although time constraints in a busy surgery may tempt the GP to avoid investing a large amount of time in an often unplanned consultation, the benefits of a thorough history, examination and pertinent investigations are manifold.

Assessment of the drug user

Elicit from the history	*Note on examination*	*Investigate*
What drug(s) are used?	General	Urine
How much drug is used?	Undue drowsiness	Drugs of abuse?
Frequency of use?	High arousal	Full blood count
Route of administration?	Signs of withdrawal	Anaemia?
(? Sharing injecting	Self-neglect	Raised MCV?
equipment)		Liver function
Duration of use?	Height/weight	Gamma GT?
Previous treatment?		Other enzymes?
Current health	Skin	Hepatitis A/B
problems?	Abscesses	Antibodies?
Past medical history?	Injecting sites	Carrier status?
Abscesses/cellulitis	Venous ulcers	Non-immune ?
Hepatitis	Anaemia	
Bacterial endocarditis	Parasites	Consider:
Septicaemia	Self-mutilation	CXR
Deep venous		Counselling and
thrombosis	Chest	screening for HIV,
Tuberculosis	Chest infections	hepatitis C, HCV
HIV	Cardiac murmurs	RNA
Venous ulcers	Wheeze	Pregnancy testing if
Social circumstances?		amenorrhoea is
Accommodation	Abdomen	present
Employment/income	Hepatomegaly	
Family/social	Splenomegaly	Cervical cytology
support	Constipation	STD screening
Legal difficulties	Pregnancy	
Vaccinated hepatitis	Groin sinuses	
A/B?		
Safe sex?		
Contraception?		

Adapted from Kemp K and Orr M (1996) Managing drug misusers – a guide. *Practitioner*. **240**: 326–34.

- Many intravenous drug abusers have chequered medical and social histories with frequent previous changes of GP and address. Medical records 'following' such patients can at best be incomplete and at worst unobtainable.
- A history of drug-taking activity and the patient's past and current medical problems can help to determine the most appropriate treatment options as well as enabling the detection of significant ill health.
- A baseline of the patient's current health can be established from which future deviations may alert the GP to the development of new disease processes.
- A careful medical assessment can provide the opportunity to discuss HIV and hepatitis screening and offer appropriate immunisations.
- A thorough assessment of the substance misuser's health and lifestyle demonstrates interest in the patient and may help to dispel the fear of rejection that many drug users anticipate from health professionals.[7]

A comprehensive assessment can be done over several consultations if necessary, particularly if the patient is returning to the surgery regularly for substitute prescribing.

■ Clinical examination

Drug users may not immediately declare their illicit drug use to the GP. Some fear judgemental attitudes or breach of their confidentiality or are ashamed of their habit. Consequently the diagnosis of drug misuse may not be considered until physical examination is undertaken. Intoxication with drugs or alcohol, poor levels of general education, lack of awareness of the possible causes of their ill health and reticence born of mistrust can conspire to make some drug abusers poor historians whose symptomatology is at best vague and not uncommonly masked by the substances they are abusing. Clinical examination of any substance misuser (suspected or declared) is therefore of paramount importance and is often more illuminating than the history. In addition to those observations which a doctor routinely notes during examination of any patient, it may be helpful to consider the following points when examining a known or suspected drug abuser.

■ General state

- Look for evidence of withdrawal from opiates such as increased lacrimation, rhinorrhoea, sweating, piloerection, dilated pupils and raised blood pressure.
- Conversely, undue drowsiness and pinpoint pupils may indicate very recent opiate use.
- Agitation or high arousal may indicate stimulant use, withdrawal from opiates or alcohol misuse.
- Self-neglect and homelessness are common in those heavily addicted to drugs and patients may often appear unkempt.
- Cocaine, amphetamines and alcoholism can cause anorexia and their use may result in significant weight loss.
- Generalised lymphadenopathy may be present in HIV-positive patients;

localised lymphadenopathy may occur in tuberculosis and abscesses.
- Pyrexia above 38°C may indicate the presence of significant underlying infection and septicaemia should be considered in those injecting drug users in whom no other discernible cause for fever is found.

■ Examination of the skin

- This may reveal the presence of stigmata such as scars from old abscesses and 'track-marks'. The latter appear as discolourations of the skin overlying commonly used injection sites and are pathognomonic of intravenous drug use.
- Localised abscesses, cellulitis and superficial thrombophlebitis are all commonly observed on inspection of the skin in injecting drug users and may provide important clues as to the source of sepsis in those patients presenting with generalised septicaemia, acute endocarditis or bone and joint infections.
- Stimulant use (cocaine and amphetamines) may produce significant pruritus and sometimes formication with consequent excoriation of the skin at which patients constantly 'pick'.
- Venous ulceration and/or oedema of the lower limbs is often seen and may be caused by chronic venous insufficiency resulting from recurrent deep venous thromboses.
- Inspection of injecting sites can be helpful and may reveal the presence of sinuses (commonly found over the femoral veins in those injecting into the groin) which can provide potential sources of infection.
- Palmar erythema and spider telangiectasia may be present in those patients with liver disease and jaundice may be noted in patients with acute hepatitis A or B or in those with liver failure secondary to chronic active hepatitis (acute hepatitis C rarely causes jaundice).
- Rashes may more commonly be attributable to parasites such as scabies but the presence of a diffuse maculopapular rash in an unwell intravenous drug user should alert the GP to the possibility of a seroconversion illness associated with exposure to HIV.
- Transient skin rashes may also occur in the prodromal phase of hepatitis B.
- Small areas of infarcted skin may result from crack/cocaine use[8] and bacterial endocarditis can produce splinter haemorrhages under the fingernails and petechial haemorrhages in the skin and mucous membranes.
- Scarring from self-mutilation is frequently seen, reflecting the high incidence of psychiatric co-morbidity amongst substance misusers.

■ Assessment of the chest and cardiovascular system

Examination of the chest and cardiovascular system in the sick intravenous drug user may provide a variety of useful diagnostic signs associated with any of the following conditions.

- Most intravenous drug users smoke cigarettes and the incidence of bronchitis, obstructive airways disease and tumours of the lung is higher than average.
- Intravenous drug users also have an increased incidence of bacterial pneumonia and tuberculosis. (It is worth noting that drug users on antituberculous therapy may metabolise their methadone more rapidly as such antibiotics commonly induce hepatic enzymes. It may thus be necessary to significantly increase the daily dose of methadone for the duration of the TB treatment, tapering it down again once the antibiotics are stopped.)
- HIV-positive drug users are particularly susceptible not only to bacterial pneumonia and tuberculosis but also to opportunistic chest infections such as *Pneumocystis pneumoniae*.
- Inhalation of cocaine has been associated with atelectasis, alveolar haemorrhage and pulmonary oedema and may provoke constriction of the coronary arteries, producing anginal symptoms.
- Both cocaine and amphetamine abuse can cause tachycardia and arrhythmias.
- Injecting drug users may also develop pneumothoraces, pulmonary emboli, bacterial endocarditis and aspiration pneumonias.

A cardiac murmur in an unwell intravenous drug user should be seen as suspicious and investigated accordingly. The GP's threshold for arranging a chest X-ray should be suitably low if any significant chest infection is suspected.

■ Abdominal examination

- Palpation of the abdomen often demonstrates the presence of constipation in heroin or methadone users since opiates reduce gut motility.
- Hepatic enlargement may indicate an acute hepatitis or heavy alcohol intake.
- An enlarged spleen can occur during seroconversion following exposure to the HIV virus, is commonly found in bacterial endocarditis and may be present in the early stages of hepatitis.
- Epigastric tenderness may indicate acute gastritits or peptic ulceration, both of which occur more commonly in substance misusers who may ingest large quantities of alcohol, smoke heavily and have poor eating habits.
- Pancreatitis, both acute and chronic, may produce few symptoms other than vague abdominal pain and nausea but is not uncommon amongst drug abusers who also abuse alcohol.
- Lower abdominal tenderness in female drug users may indicate pelvic inflammatory disease. Occasionally abdominal palpation reveals a gravid uterus in an amenorrhoeic drug user who has not suspected that she is pregnant.

■ Musculoskeletal system

- Injecting drug users frequently complain of muscular aches and pains, arthralgia and bone pain.
- Sometimes these symptoms are manifestations of the withdrawal syndrome but it should be remembered that the prodromal phases of hepatitis A and B can produce similar symptomatology, as can bacterial endocarditis.

- Septic arthritis and infective osteomyelitis occur more commonly in those who inject drugs.
- Rhabdomyolysis has been reported secondary to both heroin and cocaine use but is relatively rare.
- Necrotising fasciitis may present with severe and seemingly inexplicable pain in the muscles and soft tissues prior to the onset of necrosis.

■ Central nervous system

- Many substance misusers report 'fits' and the incidence of epileptiform seizures is increased in patients withdrawing from both benzodiazepines and alcohol. Convulsions may also occur in association with cocaine toxicity. True idiopathic or inherent epilepsy should nevertheless be excluded. Anticonvulsants may be used prophylactically in patients undergoing detoxification from benzodiazepines and alcohol but should not need to be continued once the process is complete.
- Cerebral abscesses resulting from septic emboli and candida ophthalmitis (the latter often presenting as a painful red eye) also occur more frequently in those injecting drugs. Candida ophthalmitis can cause blindness if not recognised and treated. For this reason, injecting drug users with a conjunctivitis which does not clear within three days of chloramphenicol treatment should be referred to ophthalmology for urgent assessment.
- Peripheral neuropathy may be noted in chronic alcohol abusers and may also result from the inhalation of volatile substances such as butane.
- HIV-positive substance misusers may also present with cerebral toxoplasmosis, cryptococcal meningitis, cerebral lymphoma or any other of the well-documented neurological manifestations associated with HIV infection.

■ Special problems of women drug users

Many women support their drug habit by prostitution and are therefore at greater risk of contracting chlamydia, gonorrhoea and other sexually transmitted diseases. Even those women not 'street-working' are at increased risk of venereal diseases because safer sexual practices are not widespread amongst drug users. Pelvic examination, high vaginal and endocervical swabs should be performed in female drug users complaining of vaginal discharge, lower abdominal pain or urinary tract symptoms. Referral to a genitourinary medicine clinic can be offered (and provides invaluable help with contact tracing should this be neccessary), although not all patients will accept this and even those who do will not always attend once such appointments are made.

Both prostitution and the increased prevalence of HIV amongst intravenous drug users significantly increase the risk of cervical intraepithelial neoplasia (CIN) in women who abuse drugs.[9] Human papilloma virus and herpes virus are also more commonly found in drug users. Cervical cytological screening therefore reveals a much higher incidence of abnormalities amongst substance misusers and it is worthwhile performing a smear on all female drug users as part of an overall health assessment. Although some patients will express anxiety about pelvic examination (there is extensive research establishing a high incidence of childhood sexual abuse amongst drug users), it should be remembered that the drug user's often peripatetic lifestyle and irregular contact with medical services means that she is much more likely to slip through the conventional screening net.

■ Contraception

Contraception can also be discussed during sexual health screening. A large number of female patients using opiates will complain of amenorrhoea and many of these will assume that they are therefore infertile and do not require contraception. The increased prevalence of hepatitis B and C (and associated liver damage), alcohol abuse, tuberculosis, HIV, amenorrhoea and history of deep venous thrombosis, combined with the chaotic lifestyles sometimes observed in intravenous drug users, means that the contraceptive needs of such women need careful thought and discussion.

The combined oral contraceptive pill is more likely to be contraindicated, barrier methods of contraception are less likely to be religiously used, the intrauterine contraceptive device may be less widely advocated in a group at increased risk of pelvic sepsis anyway (with the possible exception of the progesterone IUCD) and the progesterone-only pill may have an unacceptably high failure rate. Progesterone implants may be of value to those patients who are able to return for their removal but not all patients wish to accept their long half-life or the necessity of surgical implantation and removal. Injectable methods of contraception (such as depot medroxyprogesterone acetate) have much to offer in that they are generally believed to be non-toxic to the liver, have a negligible failure rate providing that they are given when due, are convenient in that they are non-intercourse related and do not require a daily 'routine'. However, there is at least a theoretical risk that they may induce or aggravate osteoporosis in those patients who already are or may become amenorrhoeic as a result of progesterone injections.

■ Osteoporosis

Osteoporosis secondary to prolonged amenorrhoea occurs as a result of low oestrogen levels and is more likely in women whose amenorrhoea is of greater than five years' duration, who are significantly underweight and who are cigarette smokers. Measurement of the plasma oestradiol level (values <100 pmol/l indicate an increased risk of osteoporosis), bone density studies or the administration of a progestagen challenge test (5 mg of oral medroxyprogesterone acetate daily for five days will produce a 'withdrawal bleed' if the patient's oestrogen levels are normal) can help to establish those patients at significant risk of osteoporosis.[10]

■ Investigating the intravenous drug user

Baseline investigations (*see* box on p. 22) are particularly useful in the assessment of an intravenous drug user's general health. Such tests can provide much information that is an invaluable aid to the interpretation of the sometimes vague history, multiple symptomatology and non-specific signs with which substance misusers may present. In addition, unsuspected disease can be identified and susceptibility to preventable diseases (such as hepatitis A and B) can be determined.

The screening of urine for drugs of abuse can provide verification of which drugs are being misused and can be a useful tool in the assessment of a drug user's treatment progress. Routine urinalysis for blood, protein, glucose and the presence of leucocytes may furnish evidence of previously unsuspected renal disease or diabetes and may provide confirmatory evidence of suspected urinary tract infection.

Blood tests can be difficult to perform on intravenous drug users with extensively damaged peripheral veins. Inspection of sites such as the posterior of the forearm (less accessible to those self-injecting and therefore commonly preserved), the back of the hands and the dorsum of the feet can demonstrate the presence of patent veins. Some intravenous drug users may offer to take their own blood samples, particularly those who are aware that they have poor venous access and who regularly inject themselves into the femoral veins.

A simple full blood count not uncommonly reveals unsuspected but significant anaemia (often due to iron deficiency) and the mean corpuscular volume is frequently raised in patients misusing alcohol. A white cell count and differential are useful in the diagnosis of acute infections. Liver function tests are often abnormal in intravenous drug users, largely due to the prevalence of hepatitis B and C in this population and the high incidence of alcoholism. Abnormally raised liver enzymes may often provide the first indication of an otherwise 'silent' but acute infection with hepatitis B.

■ Hepatitis B

Serological testing for hepatitis B markers will identify which patients have previously been exposed to the disease, which remain carriers and which should be offered hepatitis B immunisation. Hepatitis B remains prevalent amongst intravenous drug users and up to half of those screened show evidence of previous infection,[11] although many can recall no episode of jaundice. The disease is particularly virulent in drug users because there is often concomitant infection with hepatitis D.[12] Few drug users show evidence of previous immunisation against hepatitis B despite the fact that vaccine has been available since 1981 and they are at high risk of contracting the illness.[13] This may reflect the limited availability of both screening and vaccine in drug treatment clinics,[14] the difficulty that some drug users experience registering with a GP and the fact that there is some evidence suggesting that intravenous drug users may not mount as effective an immune response when vaccine is administered.[15] Hepatitis B is likely to remain an important cause of mortality and morbidity in substance misusers until effective immunisation rates are achieved.

If any group of professionals can begin to break the chain of hepatitis B infection in intravenous drug users then hope must lie with general practitioners. Vaccines available are safe, have few reported side-effects, can (and should) be given to those who are HIV positive and are not contraindicated in pregnancy. Post-vaccination serology (2–4 months after completion of a course) is needed to determine whether immunity has been successfully conferred. Patients should be offered vaccine if the hepatitis B core antibody (anti-HBcore), hepatitis B surface antigen (HepBSag) and the hepatitis B surface antibody (anti-HepBsurface) are all negative. A positive core antibody suggests previous infection with the disease and a positive surface antigen indicates acute infection. It is the hepatitis B surface antibody that should rise in response to vaccination; titres >100 IU/ml indicate successful immunisation.

The standard immunisation schedule for administration of hepatitis B vaccine is to give doses at 0, 1 and 6 months. However, drug users may be peripatetic and are often homeless and in our practice we use an accelerated schedule of 0,1 and 2 months, giving the first dose of vaccine at the same time that blood is taken for hepatitis B markers and before the result of this is known. Even shorter schedules of 0, 7 and 21 days have been implemented elsewhere and have been shown to be acceptable to the homeless.[16] If, after the third dose using the accelerated schedule, post-vaccination serology indicates successful seroconversion, a booster is given at 12 months. Non-responders (those who show no rise in hepatitis B surface antibody after a course of vaccine) may be treated by offering a further course immediately – some authorities recommend doubling the dose of vaccine. The immunological response to hepatitis B vaccination may be impaired in those who are HIV positive or otherwise immunocompromised or who are over 40 years of age.

■ Hepatitis A

This disease is also common in drug users, particularly those who are homeless. Immunisation should be considered in those at risk. An effective combined vaccine is available for hepatitis A and B in those vulnerable to both illnesses.

■ Hepatitis C

Most new cases of hepatitis C in the UK occur in injecting drug users and evidence of hepatitis C infection is found in 50–70% of intravenous drug users in the developed world.[17] Serological testing for hepatitis C antibodies requires careful counselling of the patient before it is undertaken. Effective treatments are neither fully developed nor universally available, although there is evidence that treatment with antiretroviral drugs and interferon may clear the virus and it is possible that suitable treatment will become more widely available. Unlike infection with hepatitis B virus, most patients with hepatitis C appear to remain carriers.

If hepatitis C antibody is found in the serum, a further test for hepatitis C RNA should be performed (this test may not be available to GPs in every area in which case local specialist services can undertake it, along with HCV genotyping). Up to 80% of patients who test positive for HCV antibody will also have detectable levels of HCV RNA and these patients have chronic hepatitis C. Those who do not have HCV RNA in the serum are presumed to have 'cleared' the virus and have a resolved infection, although drug users who continue to inject are, theoretically, at risk of reinfection.

Modes of transmission of hepatitis C are less clearly determined than for hepatitis B but it is understood that the sharing of needles and injecting equipment is an important factor in the spread of this virus in the drug-using population. Vertical transmission from mother to fetus is possible; the risk is generally thought to be in the region of 2–5% and probably relates to the maternal viral titre.

Patients with hepatitis C should be offered referral to a specialist for assessment wherever possible, whether or not they are in a methadone treatment programme for their drug dependency. Treatment is not necessarily contraindicated in those drug users who continue to inject occasionally although regular unsafe injecting and chaotic drug use may result in treatment for the hepatitis C being deferred by specialist services until such time as the patient is more stable, less at risk of reinfection and more able to cope with the demands of the treatment itself. It is safe for patients with chronic hepatitis C to continue on methadone treatment if their liver function tests and clotting factors are normal and these should be checked every 3–6 months. Patients with progressive severe liver disease may be at risk of inadvertent methadone overdose as their liver function deteriorates; their methadone dose should be reviewed regularly and reduced if they show signs of toxicity. Serum methadone levels can be of value in such circumstances.

It is anticipated that a significant number of those suffering from hepatitis C will develop progressive liver disease[18] but there are no reliable indicators to determine which of those infected with hepatitis C will do so and most studies have been conducted on non-drug users who contracted the disease from blood transfusions. It is well documented that alcohol and co-infection with hepatitis B are important co-factors in the development of liver disease and patients should be counselled accordingly. Some patients prefer not to know their hepatitis C status. Others, accepting that they are likely to harbour the virus anyway, choose to be tested. A positive test for hepatitis C can inspire drug users susceptible to hepatitis B infection to ensure that they are immunised, may influence some to modify their alcohol and drug abuse and can enable monitoring and available treatment to be offered to those known to be infected. Many patients with hepatitis C are asymptomatic and few report jaundice. Others experience a variety of symptoms including vague malaise, fatigue, abdominal discomfort, nausea and anorexia.

The Department of Health briefing paper produced in February 2002, *Hepatitis C: essential information for professionals*, is a very useful summary of the subject (available online at: www.doh.gov.uk/hepatitisc). The national hepatitis C resource centre (a Mainliners project) provides useful information for professionals and patients (www.hep-ccentre.com). The British Liver Trust produces publications which are free to patients (www.british-liver-trust.org.uk).

■ HIV

The advent of combined highly active antiretroviral therapy has dramatically altered the prognosis for those infected with HIV and the availability of effective treatment has accordingly reduced reluctance to be screened. GPs should feel it appropriate to offer HIV testing to drug users on their list but sometimes testing is requested by intravenous drug users themselves. The prevalence of positive HIV tests in injecting drug users varies across the UK. Data from the unlinked anonymous HIV prevalence programme for 1993 gave prevalence figures of 4% and 2.8% for male and female drug users respectively living in London and the south east and 0.6% for men and 0.7% for women living elsewhere.[19] An audit of HIV test requests in a large London teaching hospital found that 16% of the intravenous drug users tested proved to be HIV positive, raising the worrying possibility that prevalence surveys may be underestimating the true rate of infection.[20]

Nevertheless, figures in the UK are relatively low in comparison to some other European countries, particularly Italy, France, Spain and Switzerland. This has importance because travel between European countries is now widespread and the relative availability of methadone treatment in the UK means that a significant number of other European intravenous drug users seek help with their drug dependency here. HIV tests performed on intravenous drug users from other European countries with a higher prevalence of HIV amongst the drug-using population are more likely to be positive.

It is important that issues such as the likelihood of a positive test result, the potential social and financial implications of a positive result, the patient's understanding of what a positive test means medically and what supports are available to him or her are discussed and documented before testing is undertaken. Many drug users are unclear of the difference between an HIV test and a diagnosis of AIDS; others may ask for an HIV test hoping to be reassured by a negative result without having fully contemplated the possibility that the test could be positive. Sometimes an HIV test is requested immediately after an episode of high-risk behaviour such as needle sharing and the patient then needs to be advised that testing may not provide a reliable result until sufficient time has elapsed for the development of antibodies. A wait of three months between the last episode of risk taking and the performing of the test is advisable and provides an accurate result in 99% of cases.

Once an HIV test has been taken, advising of a definite date by which the result will be available can both spare the patient the anxiety of an indeterminate wait and allow the GP a planned consultation in which to give the result. HIV test results should ideally be given by the person who organised the test and in person. Post-test counselling can be undertaken at the time a result is given and, for those who test negative, can involve useful discussion about safer drug use or sexual behaviour. Patients testing positive will need clear advice about onward medical referral, some may request confirmatory testing and all will need emotional support. Post-test counselling of the newly diagnosed HIV-positive patient is rarely confined to one circumscribed session in which the result is given and may usefully involve other health professionals and other agencies.

■ Preventive healthcare

GPs have long assumed a role in preventive medicine and are well placed to educate their drug-using patients about safer injecting practices. It is important that patients (particularly younger drug users who have relatively recently begun to inject) are aware of the risks of sharing not only needles but filters, spoons and indeed any injecting equipment. Those patients who cannot be dissuaded from injecting should be encouraged to rotate injecting sites, avoiding the femoral veins and neck, and should be advised on how to clean reusable equipment. Overdose awareness advice is essential, as is information on how to store prescribed drugs safely and out of the reach of children. All drug users should be actively encouraged to accept screening for bloodborne viruses and should be offered education and advice on the avoidance of these.

■ Conclusion

Ill health amongst substance misusers produces much misery for the individuals themselves and constitutes an important threat to public health as the number of drug users continues to rise. The cost of providing acute or emergency treatment for illnesses that could have been prevented or at least detected at an earlier stage continues to be high. By virtue of their broad training and experience and because of their accessibility, general practitioners are in a unique position to meet the diverse needs of drug users. Many of the perceived negative aspects of treating a population of patients whose chemical dependency often remains a relapsing problem can be greatly diminished if GPs can also focus on providing general medical care to a patient group who, whilst challenging, can also be stimulating, interesting and rewarding. Few other patients provide so many real opportunities to prevent, detect and treat significant diseases and few are more in need of the services that a GP can provide.

Key points

- Morbidity is very high in injecting drug users; assessment, examination and investigation need to be thorough.
- Female drug users may have particular concerns with respect to women's health issues such as contraception.
- Screening for bloodborne viruses should be offered to all drug users and immunisation and/or referral to specialist services should be undertaken as appropriate.
- Safer drug use should be actively promoted.

■ References

1 Home Office (1998) *Drug Misuse and the Environment: a report by the Advisory Council on Misuse of Drugs.* HMSO, London.

2 Leaver EJ, Elford J, Morris JK *et al.* (1992) Use of general practice by intravenous heroin users on a methadone programme. *Br J Gen Pract.* **42**: 465–8.

3 Ronald PJM, Witcombe JC, Robertson JR *et al.* (1992) Problems of drug abuse, HIV and AIDS: the burden of care in one general practice. *Br J Gen Pract.* **42**: 232–5.

4 Rhodes T, Donoghue M, Hunter G *et al.* (1994) Sexual behaviour of drug injectors in London: implications for HIV transmission and HIV prevention. *Addiction.* **89**(9): 1085–95.

5 Cohen J (1994) Problem drug users: a problem for the GP? *Practitioner.* **238**: 715–18.

6 Gerada C, Orgel M and Strang J (1992) Health clinics for problem drug users. *Health Trends.* **24**: 68–9.

7 Telfer I and Clulow C (1990) Heroin misusers: what they think of their general practitioners. *Br J Addict.* **85**: 137–40.

8 Zamora-Quezada JC, Dinerman H, Stadecker MJ *et al.* (1998) Muscle and skin infarction after free-basing cocaine (crack). *Ann Intern Med.* **108**: 564–6.

9 Murphy M, Pomeroy L, Tynan M *et al.* (1995) Cervical cytological screening in HIV-infected women in Dublin – a six-year review. *Int J STD-AIDS.* **6**(4): 262–6.

10 Guillebaud J (1994) *Contraception – your questions answered* (2e). Churchill Livingstone, London.

11 Datt N and Feinmann C (1990) Providing health care for drug users? *Br J Addiction.* **85**: 1571–5.

12 Smith HM, Alexander GJ, Webb G *et al.* (1992) Hepatitis B and delta virus infection among 'at risk' populations in south east London. *J Epidemiol Commun Health.* **46**: 144–7.

13 Wong V, Wreighitt TG and Alexander GJM (1996) Prospective study of hepatitis B vaccination in patients with chronic hepatitis C. *BMJ.* **312**: 1336–7.

14 Farrell M, Battersby M and Strang J (1990) Screening for hepatitis B and vaccinating of injecting drug users in NHS drug treatment services. *Br J Addiction.* **85**: 1657–9.

15 Rumi M, Colombo M, Romeo R *et al.* (1991) Suboptimal response to hepatitis B vaccine in drug users. *Arch Intern Med.* **151**: 574–8.

16 Wright NMJ, Campbell TL and Tomkins CNE (2002) Comparison of conventional and accelerated hepatitis B immunisation schedules for homeless drug users. *Commun Dis Public Health.* **5**(4): 324–6.

17 Department of Health (2001) *Hepatitis C: guidance for those working with drug users.* Department of Health, London.

18 Mattson L, Weiland O and Glauman H (1995) Long term follow up of chronic post-transfusion non-A, non-B hepatitis: clinical and histological outcome. *Liver.* **3**: 184–8.

19 Department of Health Public Health Laboratory (1995) *Unlinked Anonymous HIV Prevalence Monitoring Programme, England and Wales: data to the end of 1993.* Department of Health, London.

20 Birthistle K, Maguire H, Atkinson P and Carrington C (1996) Who's having HIV tests? An audit of HIV test requests in a large London teaching hospital. *Health Trends.* **28**(2): 60–3.

CHAPTER 4

Counselling drug users

Brian Whitehead

> Counselling is a systematic process which gives individuals an opportunity to explore, discover and clarify ways of living more resourcefully with a greater sense of well-being. Counselling may be concerned with addressing and resolving specific problems, making decisions, coping with crises, working through conflict or improving relationships with others. (British Association of Counselling & Psychotherapy – Code of Practice & Professional Conduct)[1]

Counselling is an important adjunct to other treatments in the care of drug users. Unfortunately access to specialist counselling and psychological services is variable and remains something of a postcode lottery, although overall there is continuing growth in the availability of these services across the UK. There is also a plethora of self-help and change programmes available from a range of sources. The Department of Health has recently produced important guidance for the delivery of talking therapies within the NHS, both through acute psychological and psychiatric services, and in primary care.[1] *Treatment Choice in Psychological Therapies and Counselling* promotes the value of talking therapies, identifies the evidence of effectiveness for specific therapies and promotes appropriate therapies for particular problems. These guidelines are particularly intended for GPs and other primary care providers to help them choose the form of counselling therapy which is most likely to be effective for a given problem.[2]

Primary care affords many opportunities for counselling drug users, as we may be in contact with them over a number of years. GPs should be able to respond to the needs of users who present across the range of experimental, recreational, social, dependent and long-term use. Brief interventions can effect change even in those who perceive few problems with their drug use and there is a range of psychological interventions which can be useful for those in various stages of treatment for more problematic drug use.[3]

When drug users first present, the GP should always be concerned to address their primary presenting problem, which is often their drug use. Once the patient has been assessed, the drug use is under control and they are stabilised on an appropriate dose of substitute prescribing, the longer term work of defining goals and effecting change begins. Counselling aims to guide the patient towards informed choices and decisions about their behaviour. However, the effectiveness of all types of counselling depends on the patient and the practitioner forming a good working relationship or therapeutic alliance. If you as a practitioner have judgements about drug users and are ambivalent and unresolved about caring for them, they will respond accordingly and this will affect any ongoing relationship.

A counselling framework for general practice

1 Establish therapeutic alliance
   - Support self-esteem.
   - Support client competence.
   - Define boundaries.
   - Reinforce client responsibility.
   - Leave responsibility for change with client.

2 Assess according to cycle of change
   - Use the cycle of change as an active tool with clients; where are they in the cycle in relation to specific behaviours?

3 Set goals
   - Construct hierarchy for goal achievement (1 is most achievable, 5 most difficult).
   - Identify strategies to achieve goals.
   - Explore conflicts between goals.
   - Identify unrealistic goals.
   - Explore rewards for goal achievement.

■ Facilitating change

Assessing a patient's motivation and readiness to change is a central component in the counselling process. A brief motivational assessment includes the following.

- What does the patient see as the problem?
- What concerns do they have?
- What do they want to change?
- How are they going to change? What strategies do they have?
- Are they ready to change?
- How are they going to keep change going?

In order to change, people must be motivated and want to change, believe that the change is more important than not changing, that the change may be beneficial and that they have a reasonable chance of achieving this.

People engage in behaviours because they have value and meaning and are purposeful. Attempts should be made to understand this value and attachment. 'What do drugs do for you?' is often a helpful question. To many drug users, drugs are a central part of their lives and they have probably enjoyed their use for many years before problems developed. Like many people with attachment and appetitive behaviours, there is intrinsic value attached to the behaviour.

Addressing attachment is important if people are to let go of these behaviours, because that attachment constitutes the greatest resistance to change.

Change has to be consistent with the individual's values and beliefs. It is often easier to get people to modify their behaviour than to eradicate it. This is particularly important if we are working with a harm reduction and client-centred philosophy. Incremental change is important to recognise and builds upon previous changes. Global change is hard to achieve.

■ Motivating patients

Motivation can be described as the probability that a person will enter into, continue and adhere to a specific change strategy.[4] More importantly, motivation is something that can be influenced by the counsellor, whose role is not to provide advice but to target that motivation and increase the likelihood that a course of action towards change will be successful. Patients may be motivated to engage or participate in one form of treatment but not another, to work on one problem but not another. They may not want detoxification but can be motivated to reduce harm or stabilise drug use. Listen to what individuals want and provide choice.

- Work with behaviours the patient wants to change first.
- Do not force change. Be explicit about the patient's responsibility for change and choice.
- Are they ready to change? Are they talking about change?
- Suggest a cost–benefit analysis. What are the benefits of staying the same? What are the costs of changing?
- Elicit and reinforce patient's own motivation.
- What do they see as the problem? What concerns do they have?
- What will change look like? What are the goals for change?
- Are they prepared? How will they change? What strategies do they have for change?
- How will they keep the change going? What support do they have?
- Who can be involved explicitly in supporting the changes that they are making?

■ Brief interventions

Brief interventions have developed from the belief that change is essentially motivational and by examining their commitment to change and clarifying their decision to change, patients can effect change. Brief interventions are effective compared to outcomes for patients who receive no counselling and appear to have comparable results to longer term interventions.[5] The components of a brief intervention have been summarised by the acronym FRAMES.

- **F**eedback
- **R**esponsibility
- **A**dvice

- Menu
- Empathy
- Self-efficacy

■ Feedback

This usually consists of a structured and comprehensive assessment, through which the patient is given feedback. This provides them with an objective picture of their situation and allows for reflection on problem areas in their lives.

■ Responsibility

Emphasis is placed on the responsibility of the patient to effect change. The GP is only a supporter of any change that the patient determines is important. This needs to be made explicit.

■ Advice

Advice should be based on an objective assessment of the patient. Accurate and non-judgemental information can be given to them to assist them to draw their own conclusions. The GP is in an important position to provide such information to patients.

■ Menu

Patients are more likely to effect and maintain change if they perceive the benefits of change and then identify the most appropriate strategies to achieve this. They should be offered a choice (menu) of optional strategies to consider. Prescribing a single change strategy in unlikely to be as effective as the option of choice. Choice gives patients the opportunity to select approaches that meet their particular needs and situation. Empowering drug users with the freedom to select strategies also enhances personal control – if they feel that they have chosen a particular course of action they are more likely to maintain any change effect. Clarifying what is available also allows GPs to reflect upon and define the boundaries and limits of what they can provide. It then becomes evident what is required in terms of support from external agencies.

■ Empathy

The ability of a GP to express empathy is a well-recognised cornerstone of effective practice. The importance of the interpersonal relationship between drug users and their GPs should not be underestimated. Users who feel judged and unwanted are more likely to be resistant and drop out of treatment.

■ Self-efficacy or competence

Patients must be able to ascribe change to themselves and identify with the belief that they can change. Sustaining a patient's belief in him or herself is crucial for effecting change.

These six elements are the building blocks of any intervention.

■ Stages of change

Patterns of behaviour are not usually created or modified in a single moment. Rather, there are steps or stages in a process of change which represent specific tasks that must be completed and goals achieved if the individual is to move from one stage to another. A helpful model for understanding the processes that a drug user may move through is the cycle or stages of change model developed by Prochaska and DiClemente.[6]

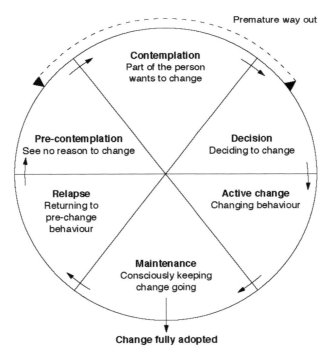

Figure 4.1 Stages of change model.

The process begins with pre-contemplation, where there is no current interest in change. A person moves through the contemplation, preparation and action stages before arriving at maintenance. Maintenance becomes the final stage in the change to new patterns of behaviour. By assessing these separate and different stages of readiness to change, the model suggests that different approaches, strategies and interventions can be used depending on where the user is in the process of change. The model can be thought of as a wheel, which reflects the fact that the person often needs to go round the process several times before achieving a stable change. Relapse is thus a normal occurrence or stage of change.

Table 4.1 Interventions according to the stages of change model

Stage	Task	Goal
Pre-contemplation – no consideration of change in the current pattern of behaviour (though someone else has recognised there is a problem)	Increase awareness of need to change; increase concern about the current pattern of behaviour, consider change	Increased consideration for change
Contemplation – an examination of the current pattern of behaviour and the potential for change	Analysis of the pros and cons of current behaviour and of the costs and benefits of change. Explore ambivalence and attachment	A considered analysis that leads to a decision to change or not
Decision – a commitment to take action to change the behaviour and consideration of plans and strategies for change	Increasing commitment and creating a plan	An action plan to be implemented in the near future
Active change – the plan is implemented and steps are taken to change the current behaviour for a new pattern of behaviour	Implementing strategies for change and revising plans	Successful action for change. A new pattern of behaviour established
Maintenance – the new behaviour pattern is sustained for an extended period of time	Sustaining change, integrating new behaviour, avoiding slips or relapse into old patterns of behaviour	Long-term sustained change and establishment of new patterns of behaviour

---

Key points

- Counselling drug users in primary care is an integral part of providing treatment.
- The techniques for motivational interviewing and brief interventions are not difficult to learn or implement and GPs are probably already using them with other groups of patients.
- Patients may require other psychological therapies at various stages in their treatment. The GP should be able to refer patients to the local substance misuse service for these.

■ References

1   Department of Health (2001) *Treatment Choice in Psychological Therapies and Counselling. Evidence Based Clinical Guidelines.* Department of Health, London.

2   Parry G (1998) Guidelines on treatment choice decisions for psychological therapies. *Audit Trends.* **6**: 110.

3   National Treatment Agency (2002) *Models of Care for Treatment of Adult Drug Users. Part 2: Full reference report.* NTA, London. Available online at: www.nta.nhs.uk

4   Sanchez-Craig M and Wilkinson DA (1987) Brief treatments for alcohol and drug problems: practical and methodological issues. In: T Loberg, W Miller and GA Marlatt (eds) *Addictive Behaviour: prevention and early intervention.* Swets and Zeitlinger, Amsterdam.

5   DiClemente C (2003) *Addictions and Change. How addictions develop and addicted people recover.* Guilford Press, New York.

6   Prochaska JO and DiClemente CC (1982) Towards a comprehensive model of change. In: WR Miller and N Heather (eds) *Treating Addictive Behaviors: processes of change.* Plenum Press, New York.

■ Further reading

• Miller WR and Rollnick S (eds) (1991) *Motivational Interviewing. Preparing people to change addictive behavior.* Guilford Press, New York.

.

CHAPTER 5

Polydrug use: cocktails and combinations, including benzodiazepines, alcohol and cannabis

Chris Ford and Tom Carnwath

Patterns of drug use in the United Kingdom have been subject to variation in recent decades. Heroin use has been steadily increasing, especially since the 1980s. Other 'downers' have become more prominent, particularly benzodiazepines. Stimulants have been used for some time, notably amphetamines. The use of cocaine and more recently crack cocaine is becoming increasingly commonplace. New drugs such as ecstasy and ketamine have also had a more prominent position in the last 5–10 years. Alcohol and nicotine have been and remain the most commonly used addictive substances. Cannabis is becoming increasingly normalised in society and is the drug of first choice of the young.

Of particular importance in these changing patterns of drug use is the emergence of polydrug use, which we define as the concurrent use of more than one drug, including alcohol. This development has been fuelled by increased availability, the emergence of new drugs and the introduction of more potent formulations of traditional drugs such as crack cocaine. Drug users combine drugs, in order to seek new feelings and levels of excitement, to heighten the experience of the primary drug or sometimes to reduce its negative effects.

■ Common cocktails: recreational use

Illegal drugs are often taken recreationally in combination to increase their effects. There is some possibility that people using one drug can predict its effect but this becomes more difficult when they are taken in combination. The risks become much harder to define.

■ Crack cocaine and heroin

This is now a very common combination, often injected and called 'speedballing' or 'snowballing'. Taken together, the effects of the two drugs are potentiated, as are the risks, especially of heart attack and overdose. Heroin is also used as a comedown medicine after crack and sometimes crack users develop a heroin habit in this way.

■ Cocaine and benzodiazepines/alcohol

These are often taken to reduce the comedown after cocaine / crack but may have confusing effects. Some users find alcohol mellows off the cocaine experience.

■ Heroin/methadone/benzodiazepines/alcohol

These are all respiratory suppressants and therefore increase the risk of overdose – see later.

■ Other combinations used

- Ecstasy and alcohol or amphetamines or cannabis.
- Amphetamines and heroin or benzodiazepines or alcohol.
- Ketamine and ecstasy or benzodiazepines.

■ **Polydrug use: dependent use**

Using combinations of drugs is rapidly becoming the norm in those seeking treatment and those in treatment. It is uncertain whether this is a new phenomenon or whether those of us working with drug users have an increased awareness of polydrug use.

■ Dangers

When two or more substances are taken in sublethal amounts, the combination may be capable of causing death.[1] A particularly dangerous but extremely common combination is heroin or methadone with benzodiazepines and/or alcohol. All can suppress respiration by different methods and the result can be fatal.

Methadone is a safe drug for opioid-dependent users when taken by itself in controlled amounts but can become lethal when taken in combination with other drugs, especially other 'downers' – benzodiazepines and/or alcohol. Often users are not aware of these risks.

■ Benzodiazepines

Benzodiazepines were first introduced into clinical practice in the 1960s. Diazepam was the first in 1963, followed by nitrazepam (1965) and temazepam (1977). They soon became the drug treatment of choice in anxiety and insomnia, as they were thought to be reliable, have fewer side-effects, be less addictive and appeared safer in overdose than alternatives. By the 1970s, they were being favourably received by patients and doctors and became widely prescribed. The high point of use of prescribed benzodiazepines in the UK was around 1980 since when it has been dropping consistently.

More recently, it has become clear that benzodiazepine use by illicit drug users, particularly opiate users, is a major problem in and out of treatment. It is likely that illicit drug users are becoming the largest group of users of benzodiazepines.[2] Up to 90% of people attending drug treatment centres reported benzodiazepine use in a one-year period and almost half had injected them.[3] They are taken because of their own effects of intoxication, to enhance another drug or to counter early withdrawal symptoms from other drugs. Several studies found that a large majority of patients reported that diazepam increased or boosted the effects of their methadone dose, the so-called 'opiate-enhancing' effect,[4] which was different to simply increasing the methadone.

Illicit benzodiazepine use

Positive effects for the user
- Cheap and available.
- Help anxiety; users feel they function better and cope with life.
- They help insomnia.
- Potentiate the effect of methadone and counteract the non-euphoric effect of methadone.
- Help with the 'comedown' from amphetamines, ecstasy, crack cocaine or cocaine.

Associated harms
- Tolerance.
- Withdrawal fits.
- Paradoxical aggression.
- Poor social functioning, 'zombification'.
- Memory problems.
- Important role in overdose.
- Unsafe injecting.
- May increase cravings for other drugs.

Methadone maintenance patients using non-prescribed benzodiazepines have been reported to be on higher methadone doses, as well as exhibiting more HIV/HCV risk-taking behaviour, greater polydrug use, higher levels of psychopathology and social dysfunction.[2] However, attending for treatment has been effective in reducing non-prescribed benzodiazepine use.

This is a major clinical and public health problem, which needs to be addressed. Users of benzodiazepines need help with this problem.

■ Benzodiazepine dependency and withdrawal

The first warnings that benzodiazepine use can result in dependency date back to 1963. The medical profession took little notice of these reports. Eventually the problems of dependence were recognised and there is now a wealth of literature on use and abuse of benzodiazepines, normal dose dependency and withdrawal symptoms.

There is a high risk of dependency and benzodiazepines are at least as addictive as opiates. Coming off benzodiazepines may be more difficult than coming off opioids. The risk of withdrawal symptoms increases with the length of benzodiazepine use. They occur in 50% of users who have used over three years and in 75% who have used over six years. Withdrawal symptoms are worse if high doses have been used but can be minimised if reductions are tapered.

Benzodiazepine withdrawal symptoms

Central nervous system
- Headache, all-over pain.
- 'Pins and needles', 'crawling in the skin' (formication).
- Weakness, tremor, ataxia.
- Muscle twitches, fasciculation.
- Dizziness, light-headedness.
- Blurred or double vision.
- Tinnitus, speech difficulty.
- Hypersensitivity to noise, light, smell, touch, taste.
- Insomnia, nightmares.
- Fits.

Gastrointestinal
- Nausea, vomiting, abdominal pain.
- Appetite or weight change.
- Dry mouth, metallic taste.

Cardiovascular or respiratory
- Flushing, sweating, palpitations.
- Racing pulse.

Urogenital or endocrine
- Thirst, frequency, polyuria.
- Incontinence, menorrhagia.
- Mammary pain or swelling.

Miscellaneous
- Rash, itching, stuffy nose, sinusitis.
- Influenza-like symptoms.

■ Control of prescribing

All benzodiazepines were classified as prescription-only medicines under the Medicines Act 1968. Under the Misuse of Drugs Act 1971 they are defined as a Class C drug. Temazepam was reclassified as a Controlled Drug in 1996 to help prevent extensive use by illicit drug users.

In England they can only be prescribed on FP10 but it is proposed to introduce instalment prescribing by April 2004. This facility is already available in Scotland and Wales.

Prescribing benzodiazepines: the case for and against

Many doctors still feel more comfortable prescribing benzodiazepines than methadone to problem drug users. A large proportion of the benzodiazepines that are available on the illicit drug scene must come from diverted prescribed drugs. The evidence for the value of methadone maintenance prescribing in opioid dependency is overwhelming. There is still no 'gold standard' treatment for benzodiazepine dependency and no such evidence for the value of substitute prescribing of benzodiazepines. There are no controlled studies of benzodiazepines prescribed in addition to methadone.[5]

Short-term prescribing of benzodiazepines may have some benefit but the benefits of long-term prescribing of benzodiazepines to drug users are less certain. There is increasing evidence that long-term prescribing of benzodiazepines may lead to increased risk taking and may actually be harmful.[3]

Possible harms of prescribing benzodiazepines to drug users

- They have street value, can be crushed and injected or sold on.
- There is evidence of cognitive impairment in those using high doses (greater than 30 mg of diazepam or equivalent) of benzodiazepines.
- They promote dependency and result in withdrawal symptoms which are difficult to treat.
- They have also been cited as important in combination with methadone and/or alcohol in drug-related deaths.
- Many people continue to buy on top of any prescription given and risk erratic or dangerous usage.
- Use of benzodiazepines in methadone maintenance patients is associated with adverse factors: poor physical and psychological health, increased injecting, increased risk behaviours, poor social functioning and worse outcomes.

Possible benefits of prescribing benzodiazepines to drug users

- Benzodiazepine use is a large problem in drug users and users may be too dependent to stop.
- Many people presenting to services have a long-term addiction problem with benzodiazepines.
- Some people self-medicate with benzodiazepines to improve anxiety and mood and to help their poor coping skills.
- Some people settle better on a combination of methadone and diazepam as a result of its 'opiate-enhancing' effect.
- Prescribing may encourage users into treatment, help them to control their benzodiazepine use and relieve withdrawal symptoms.
- Short-term (less than six months) prescribing of 30 mg or less may have some benefit in supporting drug users to control their intake.
- It may reduce alcohol relapse in a few individuals.

We can offer support and advice to benzodiazepine users so they can control and reduce their use. This does not always need to include the prescribing of substitute benzodiazepines but if it does, this should normally be on a short-term reduction. Patients must be made aware of the unwanted effects and long-term problems.

Before starting a prescription for benzodiazepines

Great care should be taken before deciding to initiate a prescription for substitute benzodiazepines. Prescribing should be for a short time (no more than six months) and with a clear goal in mind of what is to be achieved by prescribing. Before starting, it must be confirmed (through history, drug diary and at least two urine tests) that the drug user is taking benzodiazepines daily. The patient needs to be stabilised on a substitute opioid first if appropriate, have made some attempt to control their illicit benzodiazepines and clearly want to address their drug use.

Reducing-dose prescribing

This is much the preferred option if a decision to prescribe has been agreed with the patient. Diazepam is the drug of choice because it is long acting and it is harder to achieve stability on shorter acting drugs, such as temazepam. It is good practice if your patient is on daily dispensing of substitute opioids that they should remain on daily dispensing of benzodiazepines. If prescriptions have been lost or the drugs have been used before the next prescription is due, they should not be repeated.

The following procedure should be adopted.

1 Only prescribe one benzodiazepine at a time.
2 Change all benzodiazepines to the equivalent of diazepam.
3 Keep other drugs, such as methadone, stable while reducing benzodiazepines.
4 Monitor the patient carefully for concurrent psychiatric problems that may come to light as the dose is reduced.

Conversion of equivalent benzodiazepines
Diazepam (Valium) 10 mg =   Temazepam 20 mg
Nitrazepam 10 mg
Lorazepam 1 mg (Ativan)
Oxazepam 30 mg (Serenid-D)
Chlordiazepoxide 20–30 mg (Librium)
Flurazepam 30 mg (Dalmane) – not on NHS prescription
Flunitrazepam 1 mg (Rohypnol) – not on NHS prescription

Deciding what dose of diazepam to prescribe
1 Starting
   • Change to the equivalent dose of diazepam.
   • Aim at the lowest dose that will prevent withdrawal symptoms.
   • There is rarely a need to start above 30 mg diazepam daily and this is sufficient to prevent withdrawal fits whatever dose has previously been taken.

2 Divide up the daily dose
   • Keep some of the dose for helping sleep at night.
   • The patient should not be stoned or drowsy during the day.

3 Review after one week
   • If withdrawals are occurring, increase the dose in steps of 5–10 mg every 1–2 weeks.
   • Doses above 60 mg should not be used in the community.

Reducing the dose of diazepam
• If on more than 60 mg of diazepam, working with the patient, reduce by 5–10 mg fortnightly.
• If on 30–60 mg, reduce by 5 mg fortnightly.
• If on 20–30 mg, reduce by 2–5 mg fortnightly.
• If on less than 20 mg, reduce by 2 mg fortnightly.
• When down to 5 mg, reduce by 1 mg every two weeks. (NB: Can use half of 2 mg tablet or oral solution of diazepam 2 mg/5 ml or 5 mg/5 ml.)
• Users may need to be inpatients if they have been taking large doses, especially during pregnancy.
• Reduction of the dose can be quicker if there has been a short history of use.
• Reduction may need to be slower if the user is experiencing withdrawals.
• While reducing, counselling, support groups and relaxation techniques can be helpful.
• The reduction should not be fixed but titrated against the patient's withdrawal symptoms.
• All changes should be carried out working with the patient as lack of prescribing flexibility can reduce success for some patients in this difficult area.
• Reduction would usually be short term (maximum six months). This must be established at the beginning and the risks of long-term prescribing explained to the patient.

Other drugs

If insomnia continues to be a problem try all natural methods, such as herbal teas, hot drinks and relaxation techniques, before using a non-benzodiazepine hypnotic for a *short period* (+/− 2 weeks). Trazodone 100–150 mg nocte can be tried.

There have been increasing reports of misuse and addiction with zopiclone and zolpidem. They should not be seen as a safe option and should be used only in the very short term, if at all.

Who might benefit from longer-term benzodiazepine prescribing?

A few people *may* benefit from being left on a small dose (no more than 30 mg diazepam daily). These may include:

- those with an alcohol problem who have come off alcohol using benzodiazepines and who find it difficult to abstain unless they are on a small dose of benzodiazepines. However, this strategy only works occasionally. If alcohol misuse continues the tranquilliser should be reduced and stopped
- a few people who have a long-term opiate and benzodiazepine problem and do not stabilise on opiate substitution medication alone
- a small number of people who have mental health issues and/or poor coping skills who have been self-medicating.

Key points

- Benzodiazepine abuse is a growing problem.
- Most abused benzodiazepines have been prescribed or diverted from prescriptions. Overgenerous prescribing will therefore exacerbate the problem.
- GPs should be more wiling to prescribe methadone to opiate users than benzodiazepines.
- Benzodiazepine abuse is associated with a number of high-risk behaviours.
- Other drug use should be stabilised first before tackling benzodiazepine dependence.
- Some patients will benefit from a reducing prescription, if properly monitored.
- A very few may benefit from long-term prescription, but more than 30 mg/day is hardly ever beneficial.

■ Alcohol

This is a very large problem in drug users presenting for treatment, as shown from National Treatment Outcome Research Study (NTORS) data, and is not often successfully addressed.[6] It is outside the scope of this book to discuss alcohol fully but it must always be addressed in the assessment and ongoing care of drug users. Very heavy alcohol use is frequently encountered and this can pose behavioural problems, as well as compromising the safety of other drugs prescribed. This section only deals with alcohol in the context of polydrug use.

■ Problems and dangers of alcohol in combination with drugs

Excessive alcohol use is harmful in itself, particularly if the liver is already compromised by hepatitis. Alcohol is also uniquely dangerous in combination with other drugs. It greatly increases the risk of fatal overdose when taken with tranquillisers, opiates, ketamine and gamma-hydroxybutyrate (GHB). When taken with cocaine, cocaethylene is produced which is more likely than cocaine itself to produce epilepsy and heart attacks. This combination also greatly increases the risk of violence and accidental death. When taken with ecstasy, it increases the risk of dehydration. There is also evidence that alcohol increases the reward-inducing effects of other drugs, such as heroin and cocaine, and therefore makes control of the habit more difficult.

Alcohol is also responsible for much psychiatric co-morbidity. The majority of chronic heavy drinkers suffer from depression, which in most cases resolves within 4–6 weeks when drinking stops. The risk of suicide is greatly increased. Anxiety, cognitive impairment and occasional psychotic reactions may also be found.

■ Early detection of problem drinking

Although there are some very heavy drinkers, many opiate users do not drink alcohol at all and some only drink moderately. It is as important as with other patients to detect early signs of hazardous drinking, as at this stage brief interventions are likely to be successful. Hazardous drinking may develop, for example, in patients who successfully give up heroin with the help of methadone but then need something to replace the euphoria that they are missing.

The most important way of detecting hazardous or dependent drinking is to ask about it regularly, even though patients may present with misuse of another drug. This may sound obvious but often opiate-dependent patients are not asked about their drinking on a regular basis. The FAST question, 'How often do you drink eight or more drinks on one occasion?', detects 70% of hazardous drinkers, if the answer is weekly or more often. The AUDIT questionnaire has been specifically designed to detect hazardous drinking in primary care. It has 10 questions and a high degree of sensitivity and specificity. Various shorter screening tools have been devised, such as the AUDIT-PC, the AUDIT-C and FAST. They are quick to administer and pick up the majority of cases.

Abnormal liver function tests are a good indication of heavy drinking but the possibility of hepatitis must also be borne in mind. Gamma glutamyl transferase provides a more specific indicator of alcohol use, while an increased red blood cell mean corpuscular volume (MCV) provides a longer-term marker.

Screening all patients is probably not cost effective.[7] It may be better to focus on those at higher risk, for example patients with hypertension or anxiety and depression. The issue of screening is helpfully reviewed on the Alcohol Concern website, where there is also a lot of other useful information.[8]

■ Brief interventions

When hazardous drinking is detected the initial response would normally be a 'brief intervention'. This is generally restricted to four or fewer sessions, each session lasting from a few minutes to one hour, and is designed to be conducted by health professionals who do not specialise in addictions treatment. Brief interventions have been found effective for helping non-alcohol-dependent patients reduce or stop drinking, for motivating alcohol-dependent patients to enter long-term alcohol treatment and for treating some alcohol-dependent patients.[9] The framework for brief intervention is described in detail elsewhere; see, for example, the Alcohol Concern website mentioned above.

■ More intense treatment

Where brief intervention is not effective or sufficient, more intensive treatment may be required through a dedicated alcohol service. Taking methadone should not be a bar to using alcohol services or to participating in Alcoholics Anonymous, although it has been in the past in some areas.

■ Detoxification

Home detoxification may be appropriate and is usually carried out using chlordiazepoxide. It is only needed in someone who has developed a state of alcohol dependency which is manifest by symptoms of alcohol withdrawal, e.g. sweats, sleep problems, anxiety. They cannot usually manage 24 hours without a drink. The key professional will be the GP, who will undertake the prescribing required and be involved in ongoing support. The Community Alcohol Service will normally supervise the detoxification. The dose level and length of detox will depend on the severity of the alcohol dependence. Any nutritional or vitamin deficiency should be treated.

A typical reducing programme for a male (female) client would be:

- Days 1 and 2 – chlordiazepoxide 30 mg (20 mg) q.d.s.
- Days 3 and 4 – chlordiazepoxide 20 mg (15 mg) q.d.s.
- Days 5 and 6 – chlordiazepoxide 10 mg (10 mg) q.d.s.
- Days 7 and 8 – chlordiazepoxide 5 mg (5 mg) q.d.s.
- Days 9 – stop chlordiazepoxide.

Some patients need larger doses and some need a slightly extended detoxification.

For those with a history of convulsions, who seem significantly confused or who have very poor home circumstances, hospital admission is preferable.

However, the process of detoxification is itself neurotoxic and so repeated detoxifications followed by rapid relapses are not beneficial. Alcohol use generally fluctuates and it may be best to work with patients to reduce and control their use until such time as it appears that detoxification would be effective.

■ Maintaining abstinence

Maintaining abstinence is difficult. About 50% of alcohol-dependent patients relapse within three months of completing treatment. Work needs to be done to maintain the abstinence, e.g. additional counselling, self-help groups. Follow-up by the specialist alcohol service should be encouraged. This can take the form of counselling, relapse prevention groups and drugs such as acamprosate, naltrexone or disulfiram.

■ Alcohol and methadone

Although it is tempting to reduce methadone during episodes of heavy drinking, this will probably lead to hazardous heroin use in combination with alcohol. There is some evidence that opiate users with a tendency to heavy drinking are more likely to keep this under control on higher doses of methadone. Liver induction may possibly decrease methadone levels. It is often a successful strategy to increase methadone gradually provided alcohol consumption is seen to reduce in parallel. Supervised consumption allows the withholding of medication if there is obvious intoxication and thereby encourages the daily postponement of heavy drinking. Continued excessive drinking should lead to a review of treatment, with consideration of inpatient or residential care or suspension of treatment in extreme cases.

Key points

- Many drug users use alcohol moderately or not at all.
- Some use alcohol for its euphoriant effects on top of methadone.
- Alcohol use is dangerous with cocaine and with many other drugs.
- Early detection of hazardous drinking and brief interventions are valuable.
- Alcohol use induces hepatic enzymes and thereby decreases serum methadone levels.
- Heavy alcohol use can cause major management problems.
- Inpatient detoxification is necessary in some cases, particularly if there is risk of Wernicke's encephalopathy.

■ Nicotine

Nicotine addiction is extremely common in those using illicit drugs or consuming excessive amounts of alcohol. There is a mutually reinforcing effect between nicotine and heroin, so that those who give up smoking find it easier also to abstain from heroin. It is an extra risk factor for heart attacks and sudden death in cocaine users and exacerbates lung damage in crack smokers. It is one of the most harmful drugs consumed by our patients but too often drug workers ignore this habit, perhaps because many smoke themselves. It is as important to offer nicotine cessation treatment to drug users as to anyone else and surveys show that they are often keen to receive it.

■ Treatment

It is probably best to tackle nicotine addiction after other addictions have been brought under control, for example after stabilisation on methadone. The mainstay of treatment is nicotine replacement, which increases cessation rates by 2–3 times over that achieved by counselling alone.[10] Nicotine can be administered by patch or gum or nasal or oral inhaler. It is a substitution treatment similar to methadone but of shorter duration. It is feasible that prolonged nicotine replacement may help some as a form of harm reduction, but this has not been properly investigated.

There is no contraindication to nicotine replacement in those using other drugs, since as much nicotine would have been consumed in cigarettes anyway.

A course of bupropion (150 mg o.d. for one week, then 150 mg b.d. for eight weeks) increases abstinence rates. It should be avoided in those with a history of convulsions and in those taking stimulants, large amounts of alcohol or withdrawing from benzodiazepines. It should be avoided in patients with eating disorders.

Key points

- Tobacco is at least as harmful as other drugs, alone and in interaction.
- Many drug users wish to stop smoking.
- This is best attempted after control of other addictions, e.g. after methadone stabilisation.
- The treatment of choice is nicotine replacement with counselling but bupropion may be helpful for some.

■ Cannabis

Cannabis is increasingly smoked and is becoming 'normalised' in society, especially among the young. It is often portrayed as a safe soft drug but cannabis is even more harmful to the lungs than tobacco. One estimate is that 3–4 joints per day cause as much bronchial damage as 20 cigarettes. It can also impair concentration and short-term memory and possibly predispose to schizophrenia if used heavily during teenage years.

Cannabis plants have been selectively bred to contain higher concentrations of THC (tetrahydro-cannabinol), with the result that joints currently may contain

300 mg THC as opposed to 10 mg 20 years ago. Methods of intensive use have evolved using hot knives, bags and buckets. As a result episodes of toxic psychosis are more common and dependence occurs in at least 5–10% of users.[11]

Cannabis is used regularly by 70–85% of Class A drug users and plays an important part in many drug repertoires. For example, it may be used as a relaxing preparation for heroin injection, as a comedown medicine after crack or as a club drug alongside ecstasy. Many find it helps the insomnia that often accompanies stimulant or heroin use. It is often used in self-detoxification from heroin and alcohol. Animal evidence supports its use in opiate withdrawal. It does not exhibit significant interactions with other illicit drugs, although cannabis-induced tachycardia may play an adjunctive role in cocaine arrhythmias.

■ Treatment

A small but increasing number of primary cannabis users are beginning to approach GPs or drug services asking for help. One study showed that those seeking treatment for opiate dependence who also smoked cannabis were more likely to share needles, to be engaged in drug dealing and to report financial difficulties. Nonetheless, most did not see cannabis use as a problem and were not looking for treatment for it.[12] One study in primary care found that there was almost a bimodal distribution of use, with many people using moderate amounts (less than half an ounce a week) but with those using more often using much more (over an ounce a week).[13] A useful way of establishing the extent of cannabis use is to ask about total weekly consumption which relates to purchasing habits. Attention can be targeted on those in the heavy use group or who show signs of dependence or physical or mental morbidity.

Medication has little part to play in the treatment of cannabis use, although a brief course of benzodiazepines may be useful for dependent users during withdrawal. The main role of a GP is to enquire about cannabis use and to raise awareness of the potential dangers, particularly in heavy users.

Standard motivational techniques can be used or referral to drug services where appropriate. A recent study showed that after brief training, GPs were able to detect cannabis abuse more frequently and to use motivational skills successfully to increase engagement in treatment.[14]

Key points

- Cannabis joints are much stronger than they used to be and therefore psychiatric symptoms and dependence are more common.
- Cannabis and tobacco cause more bronchial damage than tobacco alone.
- Opiate users who use cannabis may be less stable than those who do not.
- Heavy users use an ounce or more per week and differ significantly from moderate users.
- GPs can learn to detect harmful cannabis use and to use motivational skills to increase engagement in treatment.

■ How can we successfully manage poly-drug use in a primary care service?

- Accessibility – not excluding polydrug users.
- Include substitute prescribing and non-prescribing options.
- Staff trained to deal with the person, not the drug.
- Need to use multidisciplinary working.
- Must provide not just a prescription but also a whole range of treatments with flexibility and understanding.
- Involve users in the development of services.

Most shared-care schemes need to change their protocols to support, and reimburse, primary care to work with all drug users, whatever they are using and in whatever combination.

■ References

1 Home Office (2000) *Reducing Drug Related Deaths – a report by the Advisory Council on the Misuse of Drugs.* Stationery Office, London.
2 Darke S (1995) The use of benzodiazepines amongst injecting drug users. *Drug and Alcohol Rev.* **13**: 63–9.
3 Department of Health, Scottish Office Department of Health, Welsh Office, Department of Health and Social Services, Northern Ireland (1999) *Drug Misuse and Dependence – guidelines on clinical management.* Stationery Office, London. Available online at: www.drugs.gov.uk/polguide.htm
4 Bell J, Bowron P, Lewis J and Batey R (1990) Serum levels of methadone in maintenance clients who persist in illicit drug use. *Br J Addiction.* **85**: 1599–602.
5 Seivewright N (2000) *Community Treatment of Drug Misuse: more than methadone.* Cambridge University Press, Cambridge.
6 Gossop M, Marsden J and Stewart D (1998) *NTORS – At One Year. The National Treatment Outcome Research Study. Changes in substance use, health and criminal behaviour one year after intake.* Department of Health, London.
7 Beich A, Thorsen T and Rollnick S (2003) Screening in brief intervention trials targeting excessive drinking in general practice: systematic review and meta-analysis. *BMJ.* **327**: 536–40.
8 www.alcoholconcern.org.uk
9 Effective Health Care Research Team (1993) Brief interventions and alcohol use. *Effective Health Care.* **7**: 1–13.
10 Henningfield JE (1995) Nicotine medications for smoking cessation. *NEJM.* **333**: 1196–2003.
11 Gerada C (2003) Cannabis and the general practitioner – 'going to pot'. *Br J Gen Pract.* **53**: 498–9.
12 Budney AJ, Bickel WK and Amass L (1998) Marijuana use and treatment outcome among opioid-dependent patients. *Addiction.* **93**: 493–503.
13 Robertson JR, Miller P and Anderson R (1996) Cannabis use in the community. *Br J Gen Pract.* **46**: 671–4.
14 McCambridge J, Strang J, Platts S *et al.* (2003) Cannabis use and the GP: brief motivational intervention increases clinical enquiry by GPs in a pilot study. *Br J Gen Pract.* **53**: 637–9.

CHAPTER 6

Care of opiate users: maintenance treatment

Jenny Keen and Judy Bury

■ Opiate dependence

Long-term opiate dependence is now increasingly viewed as a chronic relapsing condition which may persist in a disabling fashion for many years, with opiate users often undergoing cycles of drug use during which periods of abstinence may be followed by periods of relapse. Untreated opiate dependence, typically on heroin, can be very damaging to the life of the drug user and his or her family, carrying with it the high cost of the drug (often £30–100 daily), the consequent drive towards criminal behaviour to finance this expenditure, periods spent in prison and social exclusion. The need to obtain and use heroin at least three times a day can come to predominate over all other activities.[1]

Where heroin is used by injection, the preferred route for heavy users because of the relative efficiency of this method of delivery, the health risks encountered include deep vein thrombosis, pulmonary embolus and sepsis both local and systemic. Where injecting equipment is shared, there are the attendant risks of transmission of bloodborne viruses, with an estimated 20–70% of injecting drug users being positive for hepatitis C antibodies.[2] Although the proportion of injecting drug users who have evidence of hepatitis B and HIV is lower, the risk is nevertheless significant. General unwanted side-effects of heroin use include low salivary flow, leading to severe dental decay, severe constipation and adverse effects on pregnancy outcomes. Death associated with heroin use is common, with injecting drug users experiencing approximately 14 times the mortality rate compared with their non-drug using peers.[3] Death is usually the result of coma and respiratory depression from heroin overdose, often in conjunction with other respiratory and CNS depressants such as alcohol, other opiates and benzodiazepines.

■ The harm reduction approach

In response to the extremely serious consequences of opiate dependence, the relative difficulty of becoming permanently drug free for many people and the chronic relapsing nature of the condition, the philosophy of a harm reduction approach to treatment has become widespread.[4,5] This approach accepts a hierarchy of goals where the ideal outcome might be permanent abstinence but where other goals which reduce the harm to an individual of their drug use are considered valid if total abstinence is not possible at a given stage in an individual's drug-using history. These harm reduction goals could include the cessation or reduction of illicit drug use, cessation of injecting, reduction of drug-related morbidity and mortality and so on. There is now abundant evidence that many of these harm reduction goals can successfully be achieved through the prescription of substitute opiate medication on a maintenance basis.[6]

The aim of substitute prescribing is to replace the hazardous use of street drugs, which are of unknown composition and dosage and are often taken in an unsafe way, with a pharmacological preparation of known composition, taken in a safe and controlled manner.

The drugs most commonly used for maintenance are methadone and increasingly buprenorphine, both synthetic opioids with a long half-life, so that relatively stable blood levels can be achieved, avoiding both euphoria and withdrawal, when taken orally on a once-daily basis.

■ The evidence base for maintenance treatment

There is now overwhelming evidence from many studies worldwide over at least 30 years that methadone maintenance treatment is highly effective in preventing drug-related deaths,[7] improving health,[1,4,5] reducing drug-related crime and imprisonment,[8] improving family life and social adjustment and reducing illicit drug use and unsafe injecting behaviour.[6,8] It is estimated that methadone maintenance treatment may prevent up to six out of seven heroin deaths[7] and the harm reduction effects of this treatment have been demonstrated in a large number of settings including, recently, a number of UK primary care settings.[9–11] The evidence suggests that certain features of the treatment programme make a difference to outcomes, with retention in treatment being an important factor[12,13] and with best results obtained at the higher dose range.[13,14] There is also some evidence that outcomes are better where supporting psychosocial services are available.[15,16]

Buprenorphine (Subutex) is now increasingly used in the UK for maintenance treatment and whilst most studies have been carried out in non-UK settings, the evidence base for its efficacy as maintenance treatment is considerable.[17,18] Whilst there is some evidence for the efficacy of prescribed diamorphine maintenance,[19] this is not yet recommended for general practice use and requires a special Home Office licence. The use of injectable methadone in primary care is not currently recommended. Dihydrocodeine has been used widely as an opiate substitute in primary care in spite of the fact that it is not licensed for this indication and that there is little evidence for its efficacy. Its use is not recommended.

■ Why should GPs become involved in maintenance prescribing?

With the advent of improved training opportunities and proliferation of shared-care schemes nationwide, GPs are increasingly being encouraged to take part in maintenance prescribing for opiate users.[20,21] Where GPs have taken part in maintenance prescribing, the available evidence suggests that outcomes are comparable to those achieved in other settings[11] and maintenance prescribing by GPs is to be funded as part of a nationally enhanced service from April 2004 under the new GP Contract. Additionally, the 1999 Department of Health guidelines for the treatment of drug misuse and dependence make it possible for GPs to undertake maintenance prescribing within a robust clinical governance framework.[22] Whilst maverick prescribing is dangerous and should be discouraged, it nevertheless seems reasonable to expect that increasing numbers of GPs will want to become involved in maintenance prescribing, often within a shared-care framework and according to agreed guidance. Under these circumstances the provision of maintenance treatment can be highly rewarding, with drug users improving visibly in physical and mental health and well-being.

The family doctor is uniquely placed to treat a drug-using patient within a family and community context and also over a long timescale which can encompass a long-term disabling condition with psychosocial and physical aspects.

When GPs first become involved in this work, they may wish all their drug users to be assessed by their local drugs service. In areas where a shared-care model has developed, the agency then recommends to the GP what to prescribe and offers counselling and support to the drug user, while the GP issues the prescription and provides physical care for the drug user. In some areas, staff from a drug agency will see drug users on surgery premises and discuss cases periodically with GPs on site.

As GPs become more familiar with the issues and build up confidence in this area of work, they may feel able to assess the drug user and initiate a prescription themselves, knowing that advice and support from the drug agency are available. If problems arise, the drug user can be referred for further assessment or, in the case of more difficult users, have their care taken over for a while by the specialist service.

■ Assessment for maintenance treatment

Assessment should include all aspects of a person's drug-taking history (*see* Chapter 2) but in the case of assessment for maintenance treatment, the following factors should be particularly taken into account:

- the age of the patient
- the length of their drug-taking history
- the amount of drug used.

Maintenance treatment may not be appropriate for a very young person or one who has been opiate dependent for a very short period of time. In general, GPs should take specialist advice if they are considering maintenance treatment for people under the age of 18 or those who have been dependent drug users for less than a year. People using small amounts of heroin (e.g. under £30 worth daily) may wish to try detoxification as first-line treatment. On the other hand, where a person has been dependent on opiates for a number of years, is using large quantities and is suffering the health and social consequences of their addiction, maintenance treatment may well be the first-line approach.

■ Examination, investigations and pre-prescribing arrangements

After establishing that an opiate user needs maintenance treatment, the following examination and investigations should be carried out.

- Examination for general and drug-related health problems.
- Examination of injection sites, including femoral sites, to establish a baseline.
- Testing for presence of opiates (most commonly by urinalysis but saliva or buccal transudate may also be used).
- Arrangements should be made for blood testing for bloodborne viruses and liver function tests, especially if buprenorphine is to be used, although these need not be carried out before treatment begins.
- Identification and contact with a local pharmacist of the patient's choice who will be responsible for dispensing the prescription.
- The appropriate notification form should be sent to the Regional Drug Misuse Database.

It is rarely if ever necessary to start prescribing maintenance medication at the assessment visit and a prescription for maintenance medication should never be commenced in the absence of a positive reading for opiates in a body fluid sample. Although this may be possible at the first visit if an instant (e.g. dipstick) test for presence for opiates is available, it is never necessary to start a maintenance prescription under pressure or in an ill-considered way. It may be appropriate to delay the start of prescribing for a few days whilst local support or shared-care services are contacted, any relevant security checks are made (to avoid the possibility of double scripting), arrangements are made with a dispensing pharmacy and so on. The framework is thus established for prescribing to occur within a well-supported and safe environment which benefits both the drug user and the prescriber.

■ The drug user's goals

It is important to establish with drug users what changes they wish to make to the way they use drugs and/or to other aspects of their life and in what way a substitute prescription might help them to achieve these changes. In other words, in what way will the prescription help to reduce harm? In the light of the changes that the drug user would like to make, it is then possible to set some mutually agreed and realistic goals to be achieved within 3–4 months of starting the substitute prescription. For example, drug users may wish to reduce and stop their drug injecting or to reduce and stop using drugs bought from the street. They may agree that they wish to be intoxicated less often or that they wish to improve relationships with their partner or parents.

It is important that the GP helps the drug user to set short-term goals that are realistic and achievable. For example, it is unrealistic to expect someone who has been using drugs for a long time to come off drugs quickly and stay off or for someone who has been unemployed for a long time to find employment within a few months. If the goals are unrealistic and drug users do not achieve them, they will feel a failure and the GP will become disillusioned. On the other hand, if appropriate short-term goals are achieved, the confidence and self-esteem of the drug user may be boosted and the GP will feel that progress is being made.

Once the GP and the drug user have agreed on appropriate harm reduction goals, these can be written in the notes and reassessed after a few months. If some progress has been achieved, new short-term goals can be agreed. If nothing has been achieved, the existing short-term goals may need to be revised. If no progress is made after a reasonable period of time, that is, the prescription has not reduced harm, then the prescription may need to be reconsidered and/or the drug user may need to be referred for specialist advice.

If drug users are very chaotic when first seen, it may be necessary to establish them on a prescription before suitable goals can be discussed and agreed but it should still be made clear to the drug user that this is a short-term measure to reduce chaos. If the chaos does not lessen after a few weeks, the appropriateness of the prescription should be reconsidered.

Goals should be reviewed periodically while substitute medication is being prescribed.

■ Choosing a maintenance drug

There are two commonly used oral maintenance drugs suitable for general practice use: methadone and buprenorphine. Cautions and contraindications to these drugs are as for opiates in general and are described in detail in the *British National Formulary*.

■ Methadone

Methadone should normally be prescribed as the mixture (1 mg per ml) and only exceptionally in other formulations (for example, methadone tablets 5 mg in special circumstances such as for annual holidays). Methadone mixture 1 mg per ml is available in a sugar-free formulation. Methadone ampoules for injection are available but are not recommended for routine general practice use. Methadone has a long half-life (more than 24 hours) and, when taken orally once a day, can produce relatively stable blood levels with little euphoria and no withdrawal preceding the next dose. It has few clinically important drug interactions apart from enhanced sedative, CNS and respiratory depressant effects with other sedatives such as alcohol, barbiturates and benzodiazepines. There is no clinically apparent dose ceiling on its effectiveness so it can be used as a replacement medication even in people who are using relatively high levels of heroin. With appropriate monitoring, it can be used in people with impaired liver function and is thought to be relatively safe in pregnancy. It is also fairly straightforward to transfer from heroin use to methadone use. On the other hand, methadone's pure agonist effect and long duration of action make it particularly dangerous in overdose and some users complain that it causes clouding of consciousness, weight gain (less common on the sugar-free preparation) and menstrual disturbances.[23]

■ Buprenorphine[24]

Buprenorphine is marketed as Subutex for the treatment of drug users and comes in the form of sublingual tablets of 0.4, 2 and 8 mg. Buprenorphine has both a partial agonist and a partial antagonist effect at the opiate receptors. Whilst this makes it a relatively safer drug in overdose than methadone and offers a partial 'blockade' effect should a person use opiates in addition to buprenorphine, this also means that there is an apparent ceiling effect on its effectiveness so that transfer from higher doses of heroin or methadone is not possible without experiencing withdrawals. The maximum effective dose of buprenorphine equates to 50–80 mg of methadone. In the early stages of stabilisation on buprenorphine, people may experience problems with unwanted withdrawal symptoms although these usually settle down after a few days. On the other hand, it is thought that detoxification from buprenorphine may be more rapidly and comfortably achieved than from methadone and the opiate antagonist naltrexone can be started within three days as opposed to the 7–10 days which need to elapse before it can be started after methadone. Some patients report that buprenorphine produces less clouding of consciousness than methadone.

As a first-line maintenance drug, buprenorphine may be preferred to methadone in people using smaller amounts of opiates, those who really want to stop using illicit opiates altogether, those who are prepared to put up with some discomfort during the early stages of treatment and those who wish to proceed rapidly to detoxification after stabilisation. It is less suitable as a first-line drug for those people who are using more than a moderate amount of heroin per day (half to 1 g maximum) and it may be difficult for patients to transfer from maintenance doses of methadone in excess of 30–40 mg daily.

■ Starting a prescription safely

The aim of maintenance prescribing is to stabilise a drug user on a dose of replacement medication which is sufficient to abolish all unwanted withdrawal effects when that person stops using their illicit drug. It is, however, rarely possible to start a drug user on the optimal dose of replacement medication immediately, and some sort of titration process is required. In most cases the person best placed to recognise the dose level at which withdrawal symptoms are abolished is the drug user himself or herself and the dose can be carefully titrated upwards until this point is reached.

Table 6.1 Advantages and disadvantages of methadone and buprenorphine

Advantages	Disadvantages
Methadone	
• Mixture form cannot easily be injected	• Dangerous in overdose
• No antagonist activity	• Unwanted side-effects
• No clinical ceiling on dose effectiveness	• Slow clearance in detoxification
• Safe in pregnancy	• Mixture may be unpalatable
• Inexpensive	
Buprenorphine	
• Safer than methadone in overdose	
• Relatively safer than methadone if swallowed by children (50% inactivated in the stomach)	• Withdrawal effects on transfer from pure opiate agonists
• Faster clearance in detoxification	• Ceiling on increased dose effectiveness
• Possibly fewer unwanted side-effects	• Supervised consumption is slower due to sublingual formulation
• Blockade of heroin effect	• Take-home doses may be injected
	• Safety in pregnancy not established
	• Expensive

All drug users should be started on a low dose of replacement medication and this dose should be increased at subsequent visits. At least eight hours should elapse between the drug user's last use of heroin and the first methadone dose. The length of time between consultations should be as short as possible in the early stages to allow drug users to reach a point at which they can comfortably stop using their illicit drug as soon as possible. It should be explained to drug users at the start of the prescription that if they find they have to use illicit drugs in order not to withdraw in the early stages of reaching a stable dose, they should be extremely careful to avoid overdose, especially in the first few days as blood levels of the replacement medication build up gradually. Dosages can then be increased incrementally until the point is reached at which the drug user reports that they no longer have withdrawal symptoms on cessation of using their illicit drugs. In order to take away the temptation for any prescribed medication to be diverted in these early stages, and to enable the prescriber to feel confident in increasing dose levels until the drug user feels comfortable, all medication should be prescribed to be consumed under the daily supervision of a pharmacist at the start of treatment. It is essential to reach an adequate dose to prevent withdrawal symptoms as numerous studies have shown the failure of maintenance treatment at suboptimal dosages.[13,14]

Careful explanation of the risks of maintenance treatment and advice on aspects such as safe storage and risks to children are essential, especially when take-home doses commence. All patients should be warned of the risks of using an established dose after an interruption of treatment for whatever reason.

■ Dose induction with methadone

Methadone should be prescribed as the mixture 1 mg per ml and dosage should start at up to 30 mg for daily supervised dispensing, rising by 10–20 mg every few days until a level of methadone is reached that holds the patient for 24 hours without significant withdrawal but does not make them drowsy. Objective signs of opiate withdrawal include a rapid pulse, sweating and dilated pupils. If the methadone dose is insufficient, opiate users may feel well for some hours after taking the morning dose but will begin to feel withdrawn (sweaty, agitated) later in the day or during the night, thus affecting their sleep. The earlier they experience these symptoms, the more the dose needs to be increased. This can be done in steps. Many opiate users do better if they are on more than the minimum amount needed to prevent physical withdrawal. If users continue to feel uncomfortable on the prescribed dose or continue to use additional street opiates, the dose of methadone may need to be increased.

In cases of exceptional risk (femoral or neck injectors, people with extremely high levels of heroin use) the starting dose may be higher and increments larger but this should be undertaken with careful warnings to the drug user about the risk of overdose. When the drug user reports that the optimal dosage has been reached (commonly between 60 and 120 mg daily, but not infrequently at higher or lower doses than this) the dose should be maintained at the comfortable level and the drug user should be warned about the risk of overdose if other opiates are used on top of this. They should also be aware of the risk of increasing the overall opiate habit and the possibility of spiralling upwards in dose if additional opiates are used.

Supervised dispensing should be continued until the drug user is felt to be stable and not regularly using illicit drugs. The national guidelines recommend three months supervision at the start of maintenance prescribing but this is to some extent at the discretion of the prescriber and whilst safety should always be a prime concern, other factors should be taken into consideration such as the drug user's work and family responsibilities.[22] When a decision is made to allow take-home doses to be given, drug users should always be warned about the risks to non-addicted individuals, and particularly to children, and advised on safe storage of methadone.

■ Dose induction with buprenorphine

Buprenorphine should be started at a low dose and at a point where the patient is already experiencing opiate withdrawal symptoms, in order to avoid the possibility of a precipitated withdrawal from opiates. Patients should be advised to use heroin in the morning of the day when buprenorphine is to start and then to allow themselves to withdraw and to take the first dose of buprenorphine as late as possible that day. This may be dictated by pharmacy opening hours. The first dose should be low, for example 4 mg, but the next dose should then be taken the next morning and may be 6 or 8 mg. Ten or 12 mg can then be given on subsequent mornings until the patient is reviewed and the dose is then increased by increments every few days until a maintenance dose is reached. The maximum recommended daily dose of buprenorphine is 32 mg but many patients are stable at doses between 12 and 24 mg daily. As with methadone, doses should be taken under daily supervision of a pharmacist until stability is achieved and take-home doses can then be considered whilst keeping in mind the risk of diversion and injecting.

The long duration of action of buprenorphine means that it can be prescribed for alternate-day dosing if required.

■ Writing a maintenance prescription

When prescribing substitute opiate medication for drug users, the blue FP10MDA prescription form should be used. This enables the pharmacist to dispense the medication in instalments. (In Scotland the usual GP10 prescription can be used for all instalment prescribing.) The name of the patient's chosen pharmacy should be written in the top left-hand corner of every prescription to reduce the chance of lost or stolen prescriptions being dispensed elsewhere. If medication is to be taken under supervision, this should be clearly stated on the prescription and the agreement of the pharmacist should be obtained in advance. As with all prescriptions for Controlled Drugs, prescriptions must be written in the prescriber's own handwriting unless a handwriting exemption certificate has been obtained from the Home Office. The prescription must be signed and dated in the handwriting of the prescriber and the total dose of medication should be stated in words and figures. A typical methadone prescription might read as follows: methadone mixture 1 mg per ml, 110 ml daily. Collect Mondays, Wednesdays and Fridays for two weeks, start date: 1 August 2003. Total 1540 mg (one thousand five hundred and forty milligrams). Additional instructions to the pharmacist might read: 'daily supervised consumption please' or 'supervised consumption on pick-up dates' or 'daily supervised consumption, take home Sundays and Bank Holidays with previous dose'.

■ Continuing a maintenance prescription safely

Maintenance treatment is often long term and patients do not need to be seen more frequently than every 6–8 weeks when stable. To begin with patients should be seen every 2–4 weeks to ensure that the dose is adequate and that their other needs are being addressed. Later on in treatment it is quite acceptable to give the patient three or four post-dated FP10MDA prescriptions (6–8 weeks' supply) in order to maintain them until the next planned appointment. All patients should be warned about the risks of overdose should they return to their maintenance prescription after a period of reduced opiate medication or abstinence (such as days in police custody) and ideally arrangements should be entered into with pharmacists to notify the prescriber should the patient fail to collect their medication for more than 2–3 days. If a patient contacts the doctor to postpone their appointment where the replacement medication has been taken continuously, a further few days of script may be issued to cover them until the rearranged appointment. If patients miss appointments without advance warning it is unwise to continue prescribing except in exceptional circumstances, as loss of tolerance may have occurred or the appointment may have been missed because of a return to chaotic drug use or in order to avoid giving a urine sample. Whilst it is never a good idea to take a punitive approach, it is important for prescribers to have clear guidelines about situations like this which are made explicit to patients so that safety is maintained, consistency is seen to prevail and a doctor is not under pressure to make instant decisions on a one-off basis.

■ Length of time in treatment

Maintenance prescribing should not be dogged by constant attempts to reduce the patient's dose. Various studies have shown that true 'maintenance' prescribing is much more successful than regimens where dose reductions are imposed, which tend to lead to renewed illicit drug use and loss of harm reduction outcomes.[25] It may take a number of years for a person to develop a structure in their life and support systems which do not depend on drug use. Some drug users may never have had the opportunity to live as adults without the use of illicit drugs and therefore have a lot of catching up to do. Whilst people may be helped in developing appropriate responses to life events and patterns of behaviour which do not depend on drug use, it is often a long-term process and enforced reductions in maintenance drug dosages can simply destabilise the situation. After a period of months or years on maintenance medication, many drug users feel confident enough to initiate reductions in their maintenance dose and should naturally at this point be encouraged to move towards abstinence where appropriate.

■ Urine testing

The national guidelines state that urine testing should be carried out at least twice a year.[22] Most services would probably consider this a minimum requirement and many would ask patients to give a urine or other body fluid sample at each appointment. The purpose of this is twofold. First, to ensure that prescribed drugs such as methadone or buprenorphine are being taken and are present in the urine in situations where the patient's doses are not supervised. Second, to give the prescriber and the patient some indication of recently used illicit drugs, which enables a picture to be built up over time. Urine sampling should not be used in a punitive way (i.e. urines showing illicit drug use should not be used as a reason to reduce or stop a prescription) although it may be necessary for prescribers to return to supervised dispensing of medication in situations where illicit drug use gives cause for concern. Patients will usually be fairly honest when questioned about their illicit drug use if they understand the reasons for asking about it and urine testing can be seen as an adjunct to their reports of use.

It is of course mandatory to take a urine or other sample before initiating a prescription for replacement opiates.

■ Common problems in maintenance prescribing

■ Failure to stop using illicit opiates

The drug user will know whether this is because of persistent withdrawal symptoms or conversely for enjoyment or out of habit. If withdrawal symptoms are a problem the dose of methadone or buprenorphine should be increased. On the other hand, drug users may be reluctant to accept an increase in their prescription if they do not believe that this will enable them to stop using illicit opiates and that their total opiate use will merely increase. Within reason, it is probably best to go along with the drug user's own judgement regarding dose of replacement medication and to ensure that other harm reduction goals are being achieved, such as reduction or cessation of injecting, reduction in chaotic poly-drug use and so on. The drug user should be warned about the risk of overdose where illicit opiates are used on top of the maintenance prescription and consideration should be given to maintaining supervised dispensing so that prescribed medication cannot be diverted to fund the purchase of illicit drugs.

■ Failure to reach a stable maintenance dose

Most patients will report to the prescriber within a few weeks of starting on a maintenance prescription that their dose is now adequate to abolish all withdrawal symptoms. Because of differences in tolerance and also methadone metabolism, this dose may vary greatly between individuals and it may be necessary to go to high doses (above 150 mg per day) in some individuals in order to achieve stability. Supervised dispensing should be maintained where necessary, warnings about overdose should be given and expert advice should be taken if required if stability is not achieved on higher doses. Some individuals may not reach stability on a buprenorphine prescription because of the ceiling effect at higher dosages and if this is the case then a change to methadone should be considered.

■ Urine sample shows 'trace' or no methadone or buprenorphine

At very low doses urine sampling may occasionally be unreliable, so it is worth contacting the lab if this happens frequently. In other cases, the absence of a prescribed drug in the urine suggests either that the urine sample did not come from the patient for whom the medication has been prescribed or that medication is not being taken. The patient should be contacted and arrangements should be made for an urgent appointment at which the situation should be explained and discussed. If it is suspected that the patient has not been taking some or all of the medication, the prescription should be changed to supervised dispensing and consideration should be given to lowering the dose accordingly. Falsification of urine samples, on the other hand, should not be necessary in a service where the approach to illicit drug use is not punitive. In these circumstances, if falsification is suspected it should be treated as an indicator of possible return to chaotic drug use and again a supervised prescription should be initiated. The use of supervised dispensing for a period can allow stability to be regained and further urine samples can be taken over a period of time to confirm this. Outright dishonesty such as falsification of urine samples may be considered a reason for temporary or permanent discontinuation of prescriptions.

If medications such as benzodiazepines are being prescribed and are not present in the urine, given the lack of evidence base for harm reduction with these drugs and their potential for diversion, the prescription should probably be stopped.

■ Holidays

Detailed advice on prescribing for patients who are going abroad can be found in the national guidelines.[22] In general, the best approach is a planned one. Patients give due notice of the fact that they are intending to go away and the prescriber can make necessary arrangements. Methadone tablets 5 mg may be preferred to methadone mixture for short periods to cover holidays and dispensing arrangements may be relaxed. On the other hand, frequent last-minute requests for holiday medication may well indicate a return to chaotic drug use.

■ Intoxication

As in any clinical situation, it is not reasonable for a patient to arrive intoxicated for an appointment and this should be explained to the patient and where necessary, the patient should be offered another appointment.

■ Unacceptable or aggressive behaviour

Unacceptable behaviour from drug users should be treated in exactly the same way as such behaviour from other patients. It is never acceptable for patients to be verbally or physically aggressive to staff or other patients and this is no different for drug users. In serious incidents the police should be called and in less serious cases, as with all patients, efforts should be made to defuse the situation and to discuss the patient's concerns.

If isolated acts of intoxication or aggression do occur, it may sometimes be necessary to suspend a prescription temporarily or permanently. Such cases should, however, be extremely rare.

In order to pre-empt problems, an information leaflet or individual agreement may be useful (*see* Chapter 13).

■ Pregnancy

If a drug user presents who is pregnant or a person has become pregnant while on a maintenance prescription and wishes to complete the pregnancy, urgent advice should be taken from the appropriate local specialist, who may be a midwife or an obstetrician with a special interest (*see* Chapter 10). A maintenance prescription should not be discontinued because of pregnancy and the pregnant woman should be given advice about nutrition, vitamin supplementation, smoking, alcohol and other drug use in the normal way. Antenatal care for pregnant drug users will be carried out according to local protocols by appropriate individuals with a special interest in the field.

■ Intolerance to prescribed medication

True intolerance to methadone and buprenorphine is rare. Problems may be caused for some patients by the formulation (especially the unpalatability of methadone mixture) and persistence may be required but such problems should not be taken to indicate a need for tablets or injectable medication.

■ Multidisciplinary working

Whilst a prescription of maintenance medication is in itself a powerful force in improving the lives of people dependent on illicit opiates, there is nevertheless evidence to suggest that further gains can be achieved where other non-prescribing interventions accompany the prescription.[6,15,16] Multidisciplinary team working is discussed more fully in Chapter 14 and many GP prescribers will now be working in shared-care schemes, but in situations of maintenance prescribing the most important relationship may be with the local pharmacist who sees the drug user more often than the prescriber and can report problems such as non-collection of doses and so on. Patients on long-term maintenance prescriptions may require 'key working' at times of change or particular need or to work on particular problems. These may be directly related to drug use or may relate to other problems such as housing or childcare issues. Depending on the nature of the intervention required, specialist nurses, social workers or drug counsellors may be the appropriate people to take the lead.

■ Prevention of drug-related deaths

It is now well established that maintenance treatment prevents a large proportion of heroin-related deaths.[7] Contrary to fears sometimes expressed by prescribers, there is evidence that the prescription of methadone on a widespread basis, if carried out in a safe and controlled manner, need not lead to an escalation in methadone deaths.[26]

Prevention of drug-related death is covered in more detail elsewhere[3,26] but every prescriber should take reasonable steps to ensure that medication is prescribed and dispensed safely and is taken by the correct individual. This will often involve supervision of dispensed doses in certain situations and will require serious consideration to be given to the balance of risks and benefits before prescriptions for additional medication such as benzodiazepines are initiated.

> **The use of supervised dispensing:**
>
> - at the initiation of opiate replacement prescribing
> - at points of instability during treatment
> - where increases in dose are requested
> - where there is concern about diversion of medication
> - where there is concern about results of urine testing
> - at the patient's own request to help maintain stability.

■ Overdose

In cases of unconsciousness, coma or collapse where opiate overdose is suspected, whether from heroin, methadone or any combination of opiates, standard protocols for resuscitation should be followed and naloxone 800 mcg–2 mg should be given, intravenously if possible but intramuscularly or subcutaneously if necessary. (Naloxone is available in standard ampoules of 400 mcg in 1 ml.) The initial dose may be repeated at intervals of 2–5 minutes to a maximum of 10 mg. Immediate admission to hospital should be arranged.

Naloxone is short acting and there is a danger that patients may wake and then lapse into unconsciousness again, so close supervision is required.

Every opportunity should be taken to warn drug users about the risk of overdose from opiates, whether prescribed or illicit, and the importance of calling an ambulance immediately if overdose is suspected.

■ Reducing or stopping maintenance treatment

The main reasons for considering dose reduction in maintenance prescription or for stopping it altogether are:

- the drug user wishes to move towards a lower dose or towards abstinence
- failure to engage with treatment and no progress towards agreed harm reduction goals
- the unusual situation where a person's behaviour means that they cannot be managed within the service, either because of verbal or physical aggression towards staff or other service users or because of falsification of urine samples or prescriptions or diversion of prescribed medication.

Prescriptions should never be reduced or stopped because of arbitrary time limits on treatment or because the prescriber, rather than the patient, wishes the drug user to move towards abstinence.[25] Prescriptions should not normally be stopped because of continued use of illicit drugs, unless this is felt to pose an unacceptable health risk to the patient or it is felt that no harm reduction is being achieved. In the rare situations where a patient's behaviour makes them difficult to manage, it may be more appropriate to refer them on to a more specialised service than to stop their prescription. A return to supervised dispensing can help keep control over the situation where diversion is suspected. Where a prescription does have to be discontinued, it may be appropriate to discontinue it for a set length of time, e.g. three months, and then review the patient with a view to bringing them back into treatment.

Reduction of dosages for the purposes of detoxification should be undertaken at a rate agreed with the patient, although there is evidence that it is better to detox rapidly rather than reduce slowly.[25]

Key points

- Maintenance treatment for opiate users is a potentially life-saving intervention for a group of highly at-risk patients.
- Research has demonstrated it brings a wide range of health and social benefits.
- When carried out in a controlled manner within agreed clinical governance guidance, it is relatively straightforward and generally safe.
- Maintenance treatment can be a highly rewarding intervention for the drug user and the GP as clinical improvement is often rapid and visible and affects every aspect of the patient's life.

■ References

1 Ward J, Hall W and Mattick RP (1999) Role of maintenance treatment in opioid dependence. *Lancet.* **353**: 221–6.
2 Department of Health (2001) *Hepatitis C – guidance for those working with drug users.* HMSO, London.
3 Home Office (2000) *Reducing Drug Related Deaths – a report by the Advisory Council on the Misuse of Drugs.* Stationery Office, London.
4 Marsch LA (1988) The efficacy of methadone maintenance interventions in reducing illicit opiate use, HIV risk behaviour and criminality: a meta-analysis. *Addiction.* **93**: 515–32.
5 Bertschy G (1995) Methadone maintenance treatment: an update. *Eur Arch Psychiat Clin Neurosci.* **245**: 114–24.
6 Ward J, Mattick RP and Hall W (1998) *Methadone Maintenance Treatment and Other Opiate Replacement Therapies.* Harwood Academic Publishers, Amsterdam.
7 Gronbladh L, Ohland MS and Gunne L (1990) Mortality in heroin addiction: impact of methadone treatment. *Acta Psychiat Scand.* **82**: 223–7.
8 Farrell M, Ward W, Mattick R *et al.* (1994) Methadone maintenance treatment in opiate dependence: a review. *BMJ.* **309**: 997–1001.
9 Keen J, Oliver P, Rowse G *et al.* (2003) Does methadone maintenance treatment based on the new national guidelines work in a primary care setting? *Br J Gen Pract.* **53**: 461–7.
10 Hutchinson S, Taylor A, Gruer L *et al.* (2000) One year follow-up of opiate injectors treated with oral methadone in a GP centred programme. *Addiction.* **95**: 1055–68.
11 Gossop M, Marsden J, Stewart D *et al.* (1999) Methadone treatment practices and outcomes for opiate addicts treated in drug clinics and in general practice: results from the capital's National Treatment Outcome Research Study. *Br J Gen Pract.* **49**: 31–4.

12 Caplehorn J, Dalton S, Clough M *et al.* (1994) Retention in methadone maintenance and heroin addicts' risk of death. *Addiction.* **89**: 203–7.

13 D'Ippoliti D, Davoli M, Perucci CA *et al.* (1998) Retention in treatment of heroin users in Italy: the role of treatment type and of methadone maintenance dosage. *Drug Alcohol Depend.* **52**: 167–71.

14 Strain E, Bigelow G, Liebson I *et al.* (1999) Moderate versus high dose methadone in the treatment of opioid dependence: a randomized trial. *JAMA.* **281**: 1000–5.

15 McLellan AT, Arndt IO, Metzger DS *et al.* (1993) The effects of psychosocial services in substance abuse treatment. *JAMA.* **269**: 1953–9.

16 Seivewright N (2000) *Community Treatment of Drug Misuse: more than methadone.* Cambridge University Press, Cambridge.

17 Barnett PG, Rodgers JH and Block DA (2001) A meta-analysis comparing buprenorphine to methadone for the treatment of opiate dependence. *Addiction.* **96**: 683–90.

18 Strain EC, Stitzer ML, Liebson IA *et al.* (1994) Comparison of buprenorphine and methadone in the treatment of opioid dependence. *Am J Psychiat.* **151**: 1025–30.

19 National Treatment Agency (2003) *Injectable Heroin (and Injectable Methadone): potential roles in drug treatment.* National Treatment Agency, London.

20 Keen J (1999) Managing drug misuse in general practice: new Department of Health guidelines provide a benchmark for good practice. *BMJ.* **318**: 1503.

21 National Treatment Agency (2002) *Models of Care for Treatment of Adult Drug Users.* National Treatment Agency, London. Available online at: www.nta.nhs.uk

22 Department of Health, Scottish Office Department of Health, Welsh Office, Department of Health and Social Services, Northern Ireland (1999) *Drug Misuse and Dependence – guidelines on clinical management.* Stationery Office, London. Available online at: www.drugs.gov.uk/polguide.htm

23 Preston A (1996) *The Methadone Briefing: an easy to use reference guide to methadone and methadone prescribing for health and other professionals.* Andrew Preston, Dorchester.

24 Royal College of General Practitioners (2003) *Guidance for the Use of Buprenorphine for the Treatment of Opioid Dependence in Primary Care.* RCGP, London.

25 Gossop M, Marsden J, Stewart D *et al.* (2001) Outcomes after methadone maintenance and methadone reduction treatments: two-year follow up results from the National Treatment Outcome Research Study (NTORS). *Drug Alcohol Depend.* **62**(3): 255–64.

26 Keen, J, Oliver P and Mathers N (2002) Methadone maintenance treatment can be provided in a primary care setting without increasing methadone-related mortality: the Sheffield experience 1997–2000. *Br J Gen Pract.* **52**: 387–9.

CHAPTER 7

Care of opiate users: detoxification

Gordon Morse

■ Abstinence as a treatment option

Detoxification is the widely used term for the medically assisted process of withdrawal from active drug dependence. Although there is evidence that opiate detoxification using drugs such as lofexidine can be effective in inpatient settings,[1] there is surprisingly little evidence for the effectiveness of community detoxification and virtually no evidence that detoxification leads to long-term abstinence.[2] This has led some to question the validity of abstinence-based treatment, particularly in the case of opiate dependence, but in reality it is generally agreed that detoxification is an essential option for drug users.[1] Nevertheless, it should be borne in mind that the evidence in favour of enforced methadone weaning is very poor,[3] and further evidence has shown that the early weeks and months after detox can in themselves be a dangerous time – the loss of opiate tolerance can leave an individual open to accidental overdose should he or she relapse.[4]

Overall, the problem of substance misuse is global and massive and the strategies we have are woefully inadequate – we simply do not have the luxury of excluding any of them. Ever since there has been addiction, there have been people who seek to rid themselves of addiction. Being addicted to a different drug, albeit a (relatively) safer pharmaceutical one, is not acceptable to some users who often arrive at a time in their lives when they simply think that 'enough is enough'. There is an increasing body of evidence that methadone programmes, whilst making inroads into some aspects of health damage, may also contribute to others, notably problematic drinking.[5]

Furthermore, there is no 'maintenance' or substitute prescribing option for alcohol, cocaine or cannabis and the evidence in favour of such treatment in amphetamine and benzodiazepine addiction is poor. Being able to offer safe and acceptable programmes to assist a drug user in his or her wish to become drug free is therefore an essential part of any drug misuse service.

■ Who is most likely to benefit from detoxification in the community?

It may seem tempting to launch into a 'detox' the moment it is requested but preparation and patient selection are important. Although relapse is an integral part of the addiction cycle, repeated relapse is demoralising and potentially harmful and it is counterproductive to embark on a strategy which from the outset has a high risk of failure. Patients who are likely to benefit from a community detox include the following.

* Those who want abstinence. Working *with* patients and within their agenda is more effective than trying to steer them in other directions to *our* agenda.
* Those with good support. Drug users with relatively stable lives, perhaps still at work, and with supportive partners or other good social support. Homeless users, those living with 'using' partners or with little or no social support will probably need specialist residential treatment.
* Those without associated physical and mental health problems. Patients with co-existing psychiatric morbidity, chaotic polydrug dependence, pregnant women and others with complex needs may well have much to gain from abstaining from illicit drug use but are not usually well suited to community detox.
* Those who have been addicted for shorter periods of time (e.g. less than two years) and/or have relatively low levels of drug use.

Other patients who have long histories of addiction and high levels of drug use may benefit from a period of stabilisation before detoxification is attempted.

If a patient falls outside any of these groups, that does not preclude abstinence as a valid option for them but a more intensive programme, probably away from their locality in a specialist residential setting, may be more appropriate. There are several specialist centres around the UK that admit these more challenging drug users for a period of residential detoxification, often followed by a rehabilitation programme. Treatment may be funded by statutory drug services or privately.

■ Preparation and planning

It is part of addictive thinking to demand as much as possible, as quickly as possible, but detoxification as a spur of the moment intervention is seldom successful. Better outcomes will be achieved with careful planning for detoxification and aftercare.

It should also be remembered that detoxification is not a 'cure' – something to do to somebody then walk away. Discontinuing the consumption of a drug is a mechanical event but there is much more to abstinence than simple cessation. Recovery from addiction is a process, not an event. Many drug users have 'white-knuckled' their own detoxification without anyone else's help and relapsed soon after, usually because it was a precipitate decision and nothing changed in their lives afterwards.

Discussion needs to take place on the pros and cons of detoxification compared with other treatment options. The detoxification should be planned for a time which is as stable and stress free as possible and free of distractions. The dangers of relapse with potential overdose due to loss of tolerance must be heavily emphasised. It is very desirable to involve the patient's partner or carer in the planning process.

Aftercare should be planned. How is it going to feel? How will calls from the dealer be handled? If the person is at work, will it be possible to take some time off for the detoxification and a period afterwards? Perhaps some sickness certification may be possible?

It may be possible to engage with a local Narcotics Anonymous group which will give the patient support before, during and most especially after the detoxification. These organisations may use language and concepts that some people find offputting at first but many studies have shown that frequent attendance at their meetings is associated with more durable periods of abstinence.[6] Local Community Drug Teams may be able to provide similar support in a shared-care setting.

■ Withdrawal from opiates

Withdrawal from opiates can be very unpleasant. The symptoms vary in severity according to factors such as the type of opiate used (methadone is usually more difficult to withdraw from than heroin), the amount used, the length of use, the state of physical frailty of the patient, co-existing painful conditions and the level of motivation. This latter factor is often the most important. Some patients may experience little more than a week or so of severe flu-like symptoms, others will have a miserable period of dysphoria, depression, anxiety, pain, insomnia, vomiting and diarrhoea that can last much longer.

Many of these symptoms can be alleviated pharmaceutically. My view is that we should be aiming to make the process bearable whilst allowing the patient to face up to, take responsibility for and most importantly 'own' his or her recovery. Recovering from addiction is as much as anything else about learning to deal with negative symptoms rather than avoiding them through chemical manipulation.

There are various 'recipes' of drugs that may be used to ease the withdrawal symptoms in the transition from active dependence to abstinence. Their relative merits are not all that important. This may seem counterintuitive but recovering from addiction has much more to do with the context of a person's life and how to deal with life's vicissitudes than the relatively narrow mechanical step of just stopping using a drug.

It should be decided with the patient what sort of period of withdrawal they would like. Some prefer to start a replacement medication such as methadone or buprenorphine and reduce the dose gradually over weeks or months – the last few milligrams tend to be made of gold and difficult to let go. Others prefer a 'grasp the nettle' approach and a return to being opiate free can be achieved in about two weeks with a tolerable level of discomfort in the great majority of cases.

■ Opiate detoxification using lofexidine

Clonidine was introduced as a blood pressure-lowering drug more than three decades ago but was coincidentally found to have properties that alleviated the opiate withdrawal syndrome. Lofexidine has a similar mode of action to clonidine but was introduced specifically as a drug to aid opiate detoxification. It has alpha-adrenergic antagonist effects and acts centrally to reduce sympathetic tone. It does not reduce craving or have any analgesic action, but eases the rhinorrhoea, epiphora, hyperaesthesia and other symptoms of opiate withdrawal. Side-effects include drowsiness and dry mouth. The most important side-effect of clonidine is hypotension, with a risk of rebound hypertension on stopping. Lofexidine, however, has markedly reduced hypotensive action and is therefore much more suited to community use. Clonidine is now rarely used.

The lofexidine dosage schedules given in Table 7.1 are for guidance and are not intended to be prescriptive. The patient's blood pressure and heart rate should be measured before commencing lofexidine and again when on full dose (i.e. day 3 or 4). If they are handling their withdrawal symptoms fairly well there is no need to increase the dose any further. On the other hand, if there is evidence of discomfort and they have no symptoms or signs of hypotension then the dose may be increased.

In addition to lofexidine, it may be judged reasonable to prescribe some short-term benzodiazepine sedation. Sleeplessness is a common feature of opiate detoxification, as is anxiety. To be aware of one's discomfort through the long night hours and then feel doubly uncomfortable the next day through sleep deprivation makes a bad situation much worse.

Table 7.1 Suggested protocols using lofexidine

Standard protocol[7] (lofexidine mg in 24 hours, total dose to be split t.d.s. –q.d.s.)		Concurrent diazepam (optional) dose mg			Rapid protocol[8] (lofexidine mg in 24 hours)
		b.d.	nocte	total	
Day 1	0.4–0.6	5	10	20	1.8
Day 2	1.0	10	10	30	2.0
Day 3	1.4	10	10	30	2.0
Day 4	2.0	10	10	30	2.0
Day 5	2.0	10	10	30	1.2
Day 6	2.0	10	10	30	–
Day 7	2.0	10	10	30	–
Day 8	1.8	10	10	30	–
Day 9	1.4	5	10	20	–
Day 10	1.0	0	5	5	–

'Rapid' lofexidine protocol

Recognising that the standard protocol is slow to bring symptoms under control, Bearn *et al.* published a small study comparing rapid initiation of high-dose lofexidine with the traditional protocol.[8] This demonstrated that symptomatic improvements can be brought about more quickly whilst not causing significant problems with hypotension. The completion rates of the two protocols were similar.

Lofexidine with rapid methadone reduction

If the patient has been on high doses of methadone for some time it may be more acceptable to employ a few doses of steep methadone reduction in the first few days of the lofexidine protocol. In these circumstances, methadone could be reduced from the previous maintenance dose to zero over five days in even decrements and the lofexidine continued for a few more days. However, it should be remembered that whatever regime is used, coming off years of high-dose methadone over a couple of weeks with lofexidine is going to be uncomfortable.

■ Buprenorphine

There is increasing interest in this drug to manage detoxification. Patients on methadone may be transferred to buprenorphine before detoxification, as detoxification is generally considered easier from buprenorphine than methadone. However, because of buprenorphine's partial opiate antagonist effect, this transition can be uncomfortable. Transfer from methadone at doses of 30 mg or less should be straightforward for generalist GPs with appropriate support but transfer from higher doses may require a doctor with more specialist skills. A gradual detoxification from buprenorphine over a period of weeks or months can also be handled by a generalist GP but rapid detoxification is not usually recommended in a community setting without considerable psychosocial support,[9] such as that which may be provided by a shared-care scheme.

■ Naltrexone

Naltrexone is a very powerful opiate antagonist. It is absolutely contraindicated by the manufacturer from being administered to a patient who is still actively addicted, as by displacing the drug it provokes an immediate and profound withdrawal syndrome. Despite this manufacturer's warning, there are some centres that are now offering rapid detoxification under very heavy sedation, or even anaesthesia, by administering naltrexone. There is currently little published evidence for the effectiveness and safety of such interventions.

Naltrexone may, however, be valuable in relapse prevention (*see* overleaf).

■ Other drugs that may be helpful

- *Loperamide* may be used for the short-term relief of diarrhoea in opiate withdrawal.
- *Domperidone* is safe, has few significant side-effects and can be given as a tablet or suppository. It may be used to treat vomiting in opiate withdrawal.
- *Analgesia.* Pain is a very common problem in the patient withdrawing from opiates. Stomach cramps, loin pain and general hyperaesthesia often occur but also old injuries, back problems, dental pain and so on will become much more painful upon withdrawal of opiates and for weeks or months later. It is generally advisable to prescribe only simple analgesics that have no central action,

such as paracetamol or non-steroidal anti-inflammatory drugs. Painful conditions which can be treated should be attended to and the patient can be reassured that other pain associated with detoxification will abate in time. Hot baths, massages with or without aromatherapy oils and acupuncture may help.

■ Aftercare and relapse prevention

'Relapse prevention' is the rather optimistic title given to a range of strategies that would be more accurately described as attempts to reduce the ever-present risk of relapse. Various attempts have been made to elicit the aetiological factors that drive one person to become addicted to a drug, whilst another may use the same drug from time to time with relative impunity. The factors are probably many and complex and surprisingly, understanding them may not be all that helpful. Patients have to be encouraged into taking responsibility for themselves and their lives.

Helping a patient in this way may be felt to be outside the remit of the family practitioner but help can be enlisted. Cognitive behavioural interventions have been found to be particularly effective.[10] The local CDT may be able to provide some relapse prevention counselling. Engagement with '12 Step' groups such as Narcotics Anonymous is very useful for some individuals (www.na.org) and has been evaluated as being as useful as cognitive behavioural treatment (CBT).[11] These organisations provide support and a sense of belonging to a group for people whose previous experience is often one of abuse and exploitation by others and of isolation as a result. They can offer security where there was none and sometimes even work opportunities and new healthier relationships. The 'Steps' (of the '12 Steps') are themselves a blend of philosophy, therapy and moral reframing that encourages in the patient a sense of taking responsibility for their recovery.

Much more difficult but of great value is relocation. Although drugs are available almost anywhere, moving people away from their old haunts, where everyone knows them and where all their triggers and cues to use illicit drugs may be, is undoubtedly helpful. Some housing authorities can be sympathetic to such applications.

Naltrexone is licensed for daily consumption by patients who have been through a detoxification process and lost their opiate tolerance. The effectiveness of naltrexone in helping an abstinent patient to prevent relapse has yet to be established. The Department of Health guidelines and the product licence suggest that naltrexone prescribing should only be intitiated by specialist doctors with experience of this technique, although continuing prescribing could be managed by GPs.[12] Recently, however, the advent of GPs with a special interest and the development of shared care with specialist services have facilitated initiation of naltrexone treatment in the primary care setting.

■ Conclusion

Doctors should be careful not to overestimate the importance of their contribution when substance misusers ask for help in achieving abstinence, even though detoxification itself appears to be a very 'medical' process.

Detoxification is a highly symbolic event to the user. It is the point in his or her life where we are specifically asked for help in *not* relying on drugs, then or ever again. It is the point where, despite invariably having a past of many painful experiences, he or she wants to face up to a future without the defence that has been so damaging. Most of all, it is a cathartic transition from avoidance to acceptance of responsibility for his or her own future.

To assume that detox is just some sort of medical treatment after which the patient is 'cured' is fundamentally to misunderstand the chronic relapsing nature of addiction itself. We can help to make an unbearable event bearable with the aid of prescribed medication but our service to these patients has much more to do with our skills as human beings rather than as dispensers of pharmaceuticals.

In the last decade, many published papers have helped us to understand the factors that contribute to addiction and to relapse. In 2000, Miller wrote: '... a sense of meaning in life, honesty, hope, low levels of emotional negativity, absence of self-pity and a sense of peace ... is the elusive concept of sobriety'.[13] To help a person towards these goals is a tall order for a doctor but it is our duty to try.

Key points

- Abstinence is a valid treatment option.
- Detoxification should not be embarked upon without adequate preparation and follow-up support.
- Relapse is not a failure but an integral part of the addiction cycle.

■ References

1 Seivewright N (2000) *Community Treatment of Drug Misuse: more than methadone.* Cambridge University Press, Cambridge.
2 Mattick RP and Hall W (1996) Are detoxification programmes effective? *Lancet.* **347**: 97–100.
3 Gossop M, Marsden J and Stewart D (1998) *NTORS at One Year: the National Treatment Outcome Research Study. Changes in substance use, health and criminal behaviour one year after intake.* Department of Health, London.
4 Strang J, McCambridge J, Best D *et al.* (2003) Loss of tolerance and overdose mortality after inpatient opiate detoxification: follow up study. *BMJ.* **326**: 959–60.
5 Gossop M, Marsden J, Stewart D *et al.* (2000) Patterns of drinking and drinking outcomes among drug misusers: 1 year follow up results. *J Substance Abuse Treatment.* **19**: 45–50.
6 Toumborou J, Hamilton M, U'Ren A *et al.* (2002) Narcotics Anonymous participation and changes in substance use and social support. *J Substance Abuse Treatment.* **23**: 61–6.
7 Akhurst J (1999) The use of lofexidine by Drug Dependency Units in the United Kingdom. *Eur Addiction Res.* **5**: 43–9.
8 Bearn J, Gossop M and Strang J (1998) Accelerated lofexidine treatment regimen compared with conventional lofexidine and methadone treatment for inpatient detoxification. *Drug Alcohol Depend.* **50**: 227–32.

9 Royal College of General Practitioners (2003) *Guidance for the Use of Buprenorphine for the Treatment of Opioid Dependence in Primary Care*. RCGP, London.

10 Gossop M, Stewart D, Browne N *et al.* (2002) Factors associated with abstinence, lapse or relapse to heroin use after residential treatment: protective effect of coping responses. *Addiction.* **97**: 1259–67.

11 Finney JW, Noyes CA, Coutts AI *et al.* (1998) Evaluating substance abuse treatment process models. I. Changes on proximal outcome variables during 12 Step and cognitive behavioral treatment. *J Studies Alcohol.* **59**: 371–80.

12 Department of Health, Scottish Office Department of Health, Welsh Office, Department of Health and Social Services, Northern Ireland (1999) *Drug Misuse and Dependence – guidelines on clinical management*. Stationery Office, London. Available online at: www.drugs.gov.uk/polguide.htm

13 Miller WR and Harris R (2000) A simple scale of Gorski's warning signs for relapse. *J Studies Alcohol.* **61**: 759–65.

■ Acknowledgement

I would like to thank Dr Jenny Keen for her contribution to this chapter.

CHAPTER 8

Stimulants: cocaine, amphetamines and party drugs

Tom Carnwath

Stimulants are drugs that make you feel more energetic and wide awake. By far the most commonly used stimulant is caffeine. Caffeine lies outside the scope of this book but nonetheless it should be remembered that the problems it causes can be serious and are often unrecognised. These include psychiatric disorder, dependence, insomnia and occasionally arrhythmias and seizures.

Amphetamine is the most frequently used illicit stimulant, partly because it is cheap. Roughly 20% of young adults have used amphetamine but only 2% have used cocaine. However, amphetamine use appears to be declining slightly and cocaine use to be increasing. Methamphetamine and khat are widely used abroad but not much as yet in the UK. Methylphenidate (Ritalin) is very similar to amphetamine. The amount prescribed for the treatment of attention deficit disorder has increased and there is evidence that some is diverted and abused.

Young people attending clubs frequently use stimulant drugs. Ecstasy has both stimulant and mildly hallucinogenic effects. Recently there has been growing use of cocaine and amphetamine on the dance scene, partly as a result of fears prompted by some highly publicised ecstasy deaths. LSD use remains common. Two club drugs that have caused increasing concern recently are ketamine and gamma-hydroxybutyrate (GHB). Neither these nor LSD are stimulants but they are included in this chapter for the sake of convenience.

■ Cocaine

Cocaine is an alkaloid made from the leaves of the coca bush, which grows in the mountain regions of South America. Cocaine has traditionally been used by rich people (for example, musicians, stockbrokers and drug dealers) and also by sex workers but this has changed to some extent as the price has fallen. It has obtained a lot of political attention because of its rapidly increased use in deprived inner-city areas and its association with crime and disturbed behaviour. It is used widely by those who also use heroin. Almost 70% of those first attending drug services in Manchester now have urine tests positive for cocaine.

It has been easily available for some time in large cities such as London,

Nottingham, Birmingham, Liverpool and Manchester. Its spread elsewhere has been rather slower than was initially predicted but it is beginning to appear in rural areas and to have a significant impact in towns hitherto unaffected.

It is available in the UK in two forms: cocaine hydrochloride and freebase cocaine. Cocaine hydrochloride powder is still the form preferred by most recreational and professional users, whereas crack (freebase cocaine) is used more frequently in less affluent districts and by committed polydrug users.

■ Cocaine hydrochloride

This is the form in which it is produced in illegal laboratories in South America for transport to Europe and the USA. It is an odourless white crystalline powder with a bitter taste known by various terms including Charlie, toot, dust and snow. Initially produced with a high purity, by the time it reaches street users it has been mixed with adulterants such as glucose ('cut') and the purity is reduced to 50% or less. It is taken in various ways.

- *Sniffing ('snorting')*: the powder is finely chopped with a razor blade and drawn into 2 inch-long lines which are then sniffed up one nostril at a time using a straw or other implement.
- *Injecting*: the hydrochloride is very soluble in water and can easily be prepared for intravenous injection. It is sometimes mixed with heroin and the resultant preparation is called a 'speedball'.
- *Orally*: either as powder or in solution.
- *By application to mucous membranes*: for example, the gums, genitals or anus.

■ Freebase cocaine

This is a purer form of cocaine produced from the hydrochloride by a simple chemical process involving dissolving and heating with a reagent such as ammonia or sodium bicarbonate. Freebase used to be made mostly with ammonia and ether but now cocaine is usually cooked with baking powder in a microwave oven. This separates the alkaloid from the salt and leaves pure crystalline cocaine, which is broken into chunks ('rocks') and sold in small phials or clingfilm 'wraps'. It produces a typical crackling noise on combustion and is therefore sometimes called 'crack', particularly by the press. Users prefer the terms 'rock', 'base' or 'stone'. When made with ammonia, it is usually called 'freebase'. This is confusing, because both crack and 'freebase' consist of freebase cocaine.

In this form it burns easily but is no longer soluble. Crack is usually smoked from 'pipes' – sometimes made from bottles or soft drink cans – or else it can be mixed with tobacco or cannabis or burnt on a piece of tin foil. It can also be injected but must first be made soluble by adding an acid such as vitamin C. Injecting does not produce a quicker or stronger effect than smoking but those who inject claim that less is wasted.

■ Amphetamine

This is a general name given to a class of synthetic drugs with adrenaline-like action known as sympathomimetic amines. Benzedrine, a form of amphetamine sulphate originally sold as a nasal decongestant, was widely used as a stimulant by troops during the Second World War. A number of derivatives of amphetamine such as fenfluramine and phentermine were used as appetite suppressants.

Overall, amphetamine probably causes more problems than cocaine because of its much wider use. A particular concern is that it is the drug most frequently used when people inject for the first time and is probably therefore responsible for much bloodborne virus infection.

Because it is easily available, people use it for many different purposes. Common varieties of user include ravers and dancers; experimenters and 'prudent' users; speeding drinkers, who find they can drink for longer without getting drunk; young mothers needing the energy to look after their children; people self-medicating for social anxiety, depression or to suppress appetite; indiscriminate polydrug users; and 'grafters' who find speed helps them commit crime.[1]

Until a few years ago there were a number of areas in the UK where amphetamine was the primary drug of abuse and heroin was scarce. These areas included much of Wales and the West Country. Nowadays heroin has arrived almost everywhere and amphetamine has a less prominent role. But nonetheless, for many people it is the first drug of abuse that causes significant problems in their life.

■ Types of amphetamine

Amphetamine sulphate is the most commonly available substance and is relatively easily made in illegal laboratories in the UK and on the continent. Known as speed, whiz, phet or sulph, it is an off-white or pinky powder which has always been heavily 'cut' (diluted). The current purity rate is about 5%. It can be swallowed, often wrapped in a Rizla paper, snorted or dissolved in water and injected.

From time to time a more powerful amphetamine appears on the streets known as 'base' or 'paste'. This is a grey-coloured putty-like substance with a purity of up to 70%, though it is often less than this. It can be taken orally, smoked or injected.

Dexamphetamine sulphate (Dexedrine) is the only pharmaceutical preparation readily available, usually in the form of 5 mg tablets but also as an elixir.

Methylamphetamine (Methedrine) is weight for weight the most potent amphetamine. It has long been readily available on the West Coast of the USA and round the Pacific Rim. Known as 'ice' in the USA and 'yabba' in Thailand, it is rarely found as yet in Britain.

■ Other stimulants

The leaves of the khat shrub have been chewed for centuries in the Horn of Africa and the Arabian peninsula. They contain cathinone, which has an effect very similar to that of amphetamine. Khat is legally sold in bunches by green-grocers in areas such as the East End of London and Cardiff, where there are large Somali communities. Methcathinone ('Jeff') is a product similar to methamphetamine derived from khat. It has been a drug of abuse in the former Soviet Union but not yet in the UK. Many consider that the UK may in the near future suffer an epidemic invasion of such amphetamine-type stimulants (ATS).

Methylphenidate (Ritalin) is prescribed for the treatment of attention deficit hyperactivity disorder (ADHD). It can be diverted and abused, orally, by snorting or by injection. This is a recognised problem in the USA and New Zealand in particular but is beginning to happen in the UK as well. It is of similar potency to dexamphetamine and has similar effects.[2]

■ Clinical effects of stimulants

The acute effects are dose related and the speed of action depends on the route by which the drug is taken. Intravenously and by inhalation, the effects develop almost immediately (the 'rush') and if sniffed or swallowed, within minutes. The main difference between cocaine and amphetamine is that cocaine is briefer and more intense. The half-life of cocaine is 30 minutes, while that of amphetamine is eight hours.

■ Physical effects

These include a raised pulse rate, blood pressure and temperature and dilation of the pupils. Tolerance develops to the physical effects of the drug. Very large doses can be tolerated by regular users but on the other hand, there is an accumulation of physical effects which can lead to a greatly increased risk of death after a long binge. For example, repeated use of cocaine leads to cardiac enlargement, microinfarcts in cardiac muscle, impairment of conduction and increased levels of noradrenaline in cardiac tissue. All these factors predispose to catastrophic arrhythmias and cardiac arrest. Deaths may also occur as a result of convulsions, hyperthermia, respiratory arrest and brain haemorrhage. Stimulants also cause weight loss and insomnia.

■ Psychological effects

CNS stimulants initially produce increased energy, wakefulness, activity and an intense feeling of well-being. After a single dose these effects taper off, after 30 minutes or so in the case of cocaine. Amphetamine produces a high that is less intense but which lasts several hours. Psychological dependence can develop rapidly or over a period of time with consumption increasing as a result. In some cases a person may use continuously until they are exhausted or run out of the drug (a 'binge' or 'run'), have a drug-free period and then binge again. This is more common with cocaine than amphetamine.

Increasing use and doses of stimulants can result in a number of psychological effects. Visual or tactile hallucinations may occur. Sometimes users pick at their skin (the 'cocaine bug') or crawl round the floor picking up imaginary insects. Some develop automated behaviour, for example repetitively taking a clock apart and putting it back together. Feelings of anxiety, irritability and restlessness may lead on to suspiciousness and paranoid behaviour. Stimulant psychosis is a toxic state characterised by persecutory delusions and hallucinations occurring in a state of high arousal. Reverse tolerance may occur to these effects, with increased sensitisation over time. However, for most chronic users euphoria becomes ever harder to achieve. The majority of chronic stimulant users eventually develop clinical depression in spite of continued use.

Clinical effects of stimulants	
General	Elevated mood and energy
	Dilated pupils
	Reduced appetite, insomnia
CVS	Raised pulse
	Arrhythmias, heart attack
	Hypertension
CNS	Tremor
	Convulsions, stroke
Psychological	Depression, irritability
	Hallucinations
	Obsessive behaviour
	Paranoid psychoses
Withdrawal symptoms	Depression, craving, irritability
	Hyperphagia and hypersomnia

■ Particular problems with cocaine

Taking alcohol with cocaine is dangerous, because they react together to form cocaethylene. This is more harmful to the liver and heart than cocaine and is more likely to produce convulsions. Using alcohol and cocaine together hugely increases the risk of sudden death.[3] Sudden death is unusual among cocaine users who do not smoke tobacco.

Smoking crack can cause a number of lung problems. 'Crack lung' is a hypersensitivity reaction occurring 1–48 hours after heavy smoking. Symptoms include haemoptysis, chest pain, itching and fever. It usually clears up within a day or two. Other problems include exacerbation of asthma, pneumothorax, various types of pneumonitis and increased susceptibility to tuberculosis.

Finger, lip and mouth burns can result from overheated pipes. Snorting cocaine can cause nasal ulceration and septal perforation. Its local anaesthetic property exacerbates this problem. Hepatitis C can be transferred by sharing snorting equipment and pipes, as well as needles.

■ Stimulant abstinence syndrome

This takes different forms.

- The 'crash' is an acute withdrawal state following prolonged or high-dose use in which profound depression and craving occur.
- Withdrawal occurs where there has been regular frequent use and is characterised by fluctuating depression and lack of energy, which resolve within days to weeks.
- There may be re-experience of withdrawal symptoms if users are exposed to 'cues' associated with previous usage.

■ Identification of stimulant misuse

GPs are well placed to provide help with stimulant misuse. Many stimulant users avoid drug treatment clinics because they perceive them as catering for heroin users. In the early stages stimulant users may not see themselves as 'drug users' but rather as people who enjoy a good time. The most frequent symptom that leads users to look for help is the development of psychological symptoms such as depression or paranoia, because these symptoms conflict with the self-image which users associate with stimulant use.

Management of stimulant misuse

- Early identification makes treatment easier.
- Medication is not very useful but may help in withdrawal.
- Psychological and social support is the mainstay of management.
- Advice and information about health risks and safer routes of administration.
- Psychological methods: motivational interviewing, relapse prevention, CBT.
- Good physical care may help motivation.
- Dexamphetamine helps some amphetamine users.
- Complementary therapies may encourage users into treatment.

When users look for help they tend to go first to GPs rather than other agencies. However, before this happens there are opportunities for GPs to recognise stimulant misuse. Hypertension, palpitations, respiratory problems, panic attacks, depression and anxiety may all be caused by stimulant misuse and this, like alcohol misuse, should always be kept in mind as a possible diagnosis. The easiest way to increase the rate of identification is to make a point of asking about stimulant and other illicit drug use, as regularly as asking about nicotine and alcohol use.

The diagnosis may also be suggested by physical signs such as lip and finger burns, injection marks and nasal ulceration. It can be confirmed by urine testing.

■ Managing non-dependent use

Many people use the drugs prudently and occasionally but for others there comes a time when stimulant use becomes a problem. Much work has been done on the effectiveness of brief interventions in alcohol misuse. It is less well attested but nonetheless likely that the same situation may obtain in stimulant misuse. Early identification by GPs may well prevent the development of more severe illness.

The principles of treatment are the same for cocaine, amphetamine and other stimulants. Medication has only a small part to play. The mainstays are the standard psychological treatments used for treating addiction, in particular motivational interviewing and relapse prevention, as described in Chapter 4.

Just asking patients in some detail about the effects of drugs on their lives may itself be therapeutic. In one research study of amphetamine misuse, the control group received no treatment at all but were interviewed regularly by research workers. With this intervention alone their drug use improved considerably.[4] A more formal technique is to ask the patient to complete a balance sheet, writing down on each side the benefits and disadvantages of continued use.

Clear and honest information about possible physical and mental risks will itself be motivational. The process of physical and psychological assessment will facilitate discussion of health risks. General examination will include BP, cardiovascular system, chest, abdomen and inspection for local trauma including venous damage, excoriation from skin picking, burns to fingers and lips and nasal ulceration. Evidence of psychological disorder may be present, for example depression, eating disorder or delusions. Depending on presentation, the GP may wish to arrange ECG, chest X-ray, urine drug screen and blood tests including full blood count and liver function tests.

Six-part health check for crack cocaine users (adapted from Southwell)[5]

1 *Blood pressure*: test on entry to surgery and again after a 30-minute period of observed abstention from stimulant use.
2 *Visual check*: damage resulting from injecting or burns and other injuries linked to piping or smoking crack cocaine.
3 *Heart health check*: client asked to self-report against checklist of indicators for heart damage (e.g. palpitations, chest pains).
4 *Peak flow test*: monitor emergence of 'crack lung' or other lung irritation or damage.
5 *Weight watch*: monitoring weight loss and setting weight gain targets.
6 *Mental symptoms*: ask about depression, anxiety, paranoia and psychosis.

When patients have decided to reduce or cease use, relapse management techniques are useful. These involve helping patients realise which situations or 'triggers' increase the risk of drug use and devising ways of avoiding them or protecting themselves when they cannot avoid them. Although this type of counselling would normally be carried out by drug workers, whether at clinics or GP surgeries, it can be adapted for use during short consultations, particularly for patients with less severe problems.

Harm reduction advice[6]

- Avoid sharing equipment (snorting, smoking or injection).
- Use vitamin C for preparing injections (not vinegar, lemon juice).
- Reduce nicotine consumption.
- Avoid or take great care if combining stimulants with alcohol/heroin.
- Use pipes with heat-resistant glass.

■ Managing dependent use

Some patients suffer from severe dependence, with multiple physical, mental and social difficulties. As with alcohol, early problems may be addressed by attempts at reduction and 'controlled use', whereas for severe dependent use the only realistic target is abstinence. People suffering from severe dependence will undoubtedly require more intensive treatment and should be referred to specialist services where these are available. Rapid assessment and admission to treatment produce much better results in these circumstances.

Treatment usually consists of a day programme involving individual and group counselling, often based on relapse prevention techniques combined with coping skills training, complementary therapies and social support. US experience indicates that at least three months in treatment is necessary before a significant impact is made on the prognosis of heavy cocaine users.[7] Some will require and benefit from residential treatment.

At present specialist services for stimulant use are not well developed and, indeed, are absent in many areas. However, the government's updated Drug Strategy 2002 includes a National Crack Action Plan, which commits it to expanding treatment services.[8] Good cocaine treatment services have much in common with those aimed at other drugs such as amphetamine, cannabis or alcohol. Effective elements include quick response, standard addiction counselling techniques and general social support. It is hoped that the expansion and improvement of cocaine treatment will have a positive effect on addiction services in general, even in those areas where cocaine is not yet a major problem.

■ Medication

Generally medications are not particularly helpful in treating stimulant use. Some patients find a short course of diazepam useful for helping with the crash after stopping long-term use. If depression is present an antidepressant such as lofepramine 70 mg b.d. may hasten recovery.

Propranolol increases tolerance of withdrawal in heavy cocaine users.[9] There is growing evidence that disulfiram may reduce cocaine use by raising synaptic dopamine levels excessively and thereby making the experience less pleasant.[10]

■ Dexamphetamine prescription

Dexamphetamine prescription has been employed for chronic dependent amphetamine use and has even been suggested for refractory cocaine users.[11] This is a controversial issue as the scientific evidence for its efficacy does not exist in the way it does for methadone treatment, but there is some evidence in particular that injecting frequency in amphetamine users can be reduced.[4] It is advised that any prescription of dexamphetamine should be undertaken by a doctor with appropriate training and experience in conjunction with the local specialist drug service. It should only be considered for dependent users, particularly injecting users, as a harm reduction measure. There should be clear evidence of amphetamine use by urine testing and at least a six-month history of daily use. Mental illness, hypertension, heart disease and pregnancy are contraindications.

Long-term maintenance prescribing of amphetamine is not generally recommended but may occasionally be justified. The usual aim should be to stabilise the drug user over 6–9 months and then reduce and stop the prescription.

■ **Party drugs**

Ecstasy and LSD are still used frequently by clubgoers. There is growing use in some areas of cocaine, ketamine and gamma-hydroxybutyrate (GHB). Cannabis is also used regularly but is described elsewhere (*see* Chapter 5). The majority of clubbers will use moderately and intermittently and never present to GPs with any problem. A small number, however, will come to grief.

■ Ecstasy

Often known as 'E', it comes as a pill or capsule which is swallowed. Typically a single tablet is taken but some users may take several during the course of an evening. Recently a stronger form has appeared named 'crystal ecstasy'. It is snorted or dabbed on the fingers and swallowed.

The drug has both stimulant and hallucinogenic effects. There is a general enhancement of sensory perceptions, visual illusions and states of altered consciousness. Users describe a feeling of empathy and non-sexual affection towards others. The stimulant effects which are more prominent with higher doses are similar to those of amphetamine. The effects of a single dose last up to four hours.

Common physical effects include tachycardia, dry mouth, dilated pupils, facial muscle stiffness and paraesthesiae.

A small number of deaths have been reported in recreational users, about 90 in 15 years in the UK. This figure should be taken in the context of the estimated three million doses of the drug which are taken annually. A form of disseminated intravascular coagulation may occur as a result of heat stroke caused by a direct effect on thermoregulation and vigorous dancing in hot conditions. A few have died of the stimulant effects on the heart or from cerebrovascular accidents because of raised blood pressure. There are also recorded deaths from water intoxication when users have drunk water excessively to counter imagined dehydration.

Several adverse psychological effects have been described: these include anxiety states, depression, panic disorder, flashbacks and psychotic episodes.[12] These adverse effects tend to occur more often in heavy users. There is some debate as to whether the use of ecstasy can lead to damage to 5-HT neurones in the brain and whether this may be responsible for adverse psychological effects.

Party drugs

- Ecstasy and LSD are still common but ketamine, cocaine and GHB are increasingly used.
- A variety of different effects are produced.
- Most can cause adverse psychological effects, e.g. anxiety, depression, panic, flashbacks and psychotic states.
- Deaths may occur but are infrequent.
- Long-term effects are uncertain.

■ LSD

LSD is a hallucinogenic drug derived from ergot. It is frequently sold as 'tabs', in which the liquid is absorbed into stamp-sized pieces of paper decorated with vivid designs. It is usually taken by mouth. Effects can vary from mild perceptual distortions to a full-blown 'trip' lasting up to a day. Tolerance develops rapidly but is lost equally quickly. It can provoke or exacerbate mental illness such as panic disorder or psychosis and may be followed by flashbacks and occasionally 'post-hallucinogen perceptual disorder' which may persist over years.[13]

■ Ketamine

Ketamine is a dissociative anaesthetic which also produces perceptual distortions and sometimes a feeling of euphoria. It also interferes with co-ordination of movement and leads to a strange sensation which has been described as 'a tortoise crawling over Velcro'. This can be very disturbing for the unprepared. Tolerance develops quickly, requiring higher doses. Users are at risk of psychiatric illness and accidents as a result of poor co-ordination.

■ GHB

GHB is often known as 'liquid ecstasy', although it is in no way related to ecstasy. It is a CNS depressant which, like alcohol, produces disinhibition and increased libido during the early stages of intoxication. For this reason it is popular among 'swingers' and has been used as an agent in date rape. It comes in a bottle and is usually taken by the 'capful'. Dependence can occur and withdrawal may lead to convulsions. Both ketamine and GHB can induce coma and death, particularly if taken with alcohol or tranquillisers, but GHB is particularly dangerous in this regard. The difference between an effective and a harmful dose is small.

GHB has now been brought within the scope of the Misuse of Drugs Act, in particular because of its reported use in date rape.

■ Management

There are no specific treatments for misuse of these recreational drugs. Advice and information about the drugs and possible adverse effects should be given.

GHB dependence may require admission to hospital and a reducing benzodiazepine regime used to prevent convulsions.

Adverse psychological effects from ecstasy, LSD and ketamine should be treated symptomatically. Users should be advised to avoid the use of all psychoactive substances for several weeks at least. Persistent depressive symptoms probably respond best to selective serotonin re-uptake inhibitors (SSRIs) such as fluoxetine.

Key points

- Stimulant users often present first to GPs.
- Early detection of stimulant misuse can prevent serious problems.
- Regular health assessment can increase motivation to change.
- Dependent stimulant use causes serious physical and psychological problems.
- Amphetamine causes more problems overall than cocaine because its use is much more common.
- New party drugs are causing new problems.

■ References

1 Klee H (1997) A typology of amphetamine users in the UK. In: H Klee (ed) *Amphetamine Misuse. International perspectives on current trends.* Harwood Academic, Amsterdam.
2 Alexander Morton W and Stockton GG (2000) Methylphenidate abuse and psychiatric side effects. *J Clin Psychiat.* 2: 159–64.
3 Rose JS (1994) Cocaethylene: a current understanding of the active metabolite of cocaine and ethanol. *Am J Emerg Med.* 12(4): 489–90.
4 Klee H, Wright S, Carnwath T *et al.* (2001) The role of substitute therapy in the treatment of problem amphetamine use. *Drug Alcohol Rev.* 20: 417–29.
5 Southwell M (2003) *Crack Cocaine: assessing the problem in primary care and developing simple tools.* Presentation to Royal College of General Practitioners Cocaine Training Seminar.
6 Gray A (2003) *Harm Minimisation for Crack and Cocaine Users.* National Treatment Agency, London.
7 Simpson DD, Joe GW, Fletcher B *et al.* (1999) A national evaluation of treatment outcomes for cocaine dependence. *Arch Gen Psychiat.* 56: 507–14.

8   Home Office Drugs Strategy Directorate (2002) *Updated Drug Strategy*. Stationery Office, London.

9   Kampman KM, Volpicelli JR, Mulvaney F *et al.* (2001) Effectiveness of propranolol for cocaine dependence treatment may depend on cocaine withdrawal symptom severity. *Drug Alcohol Depend.* **63**(1): 69–78.

10   McCance-Katz EF, Kosten TR and Jatlow P (1998) Disulfiram effects on acute cocaine administration. *Drug Alcohol Depend.* **52**(1): 27–39.

11   Shearer J, Wodak A, von Beck I *et al.* (2003) Pilot randomised double blind placebo-controlled study of dexamphetamine for cocaine dependence. *Addiction.* **98**: 1137–41.

12   McGuire PK, Cope H and Fahy T (1994) Diversity of psychopathology associated with use of 3,4-methylenedioxymethamphetamine ('Ecstasy'). *Br J Psychiat.* **165**: 391–5.

13   Abraham HD and Aldridge AM (1993) Adverse consequences of lysergic acid diethylamide. *Addiction.* **88**: 1327–34.

■ Further reading

• National Treatment Agency (2002) Treating cocaine/crack dependence. *NTA Findings.* **August**. Available online at: www.nta.nhs.uk
• Royal College of General Practitioners (2003) *Guidelines on Managing Cocaine Users in Primary Care.* RCGP, London. Available online at: www.smmgp.co.uk

■ Acknowledgements

Many thanks to Dr Philip Fleming, whose chapter in the first edition I have revised. Quite a lot of his text has survived but the views expressed are my own. Many thanks also to Dr Chris Ford for her careful reading of the first draft and for many helpful suggestions.

CHAPTER 9

Safer injecting, safer use, safer sex: a harm reduction approach

Clare Gerada

General practitioners are ideally placed to reduce the potential harm that illicit drug use can cause to the individual. The surgery is often the first port of call for the drug user and his or her family seeking advice. Even if the primary health-care team is reluctant to offer substitute prescribing, general medical services, including advice about safer drug use, should be available to all patients attending for help. Whilst illicit drug use can never be 'safe', it can be made 'safer'. Advising users to use more safely is not sanctioning drug use but seeking to limit the harm caused by that use. This chapter will focus on the help the primary healthcare team can give to reduce the morbidity and mortality caused by illicit drug use and related behaviours.

■ Safer injecting

Complications associated with drug use can occur either directly from the drug itself, such as overdose, or indirectly from dangers associated with the route of use, in particular injecting use.

Complications of injecting drug use

Technique specific

- Abscesses.
- Cellulitis.
- Embolic events/DVT.

Sharing

- HIV/AIDS.
- Hepatitis B, C.

General

- Anaemia.
- Poor nutrition.
- Menstrual irregularities.
- Dental caries.

■ Drug-related complications

Drugs obtained on the street are rarely pure and are frequently cut with other substances. These adulterants are often insoluble and some (such as Vim or quinine) can be dangerous. It is also impossible for users to determine the purity of the illicit drugs they may use. In particular, injecting drug users have the least margin of error if the purity of the street drug is unusually high. Overdosage of sedative drugs leading to respiratory depression, hypothermia and coma can result. Basic advice about knowing your dealer, not using alone, reducing 'normal' dose after a period of abstinence, the correct recovery position if someone finds a friend unconscious and immediate summoning of an ambulance can save lives. Equipping injecting opiate users with preloaded syringes of naloxone may be the greatest harm reduction intervention a general practitioner can make. This intervention is not currently in practice but is worth debate despite obvious controversies.[1]

Though heroin is the drug most often associated with injecting use, almost all other commonly abused drugs can be injected, either in a form designed for parenteral use, by crushing tablets or by injecting the oral liquid formulation directly. If the substance injected has not fully dissolved or if the liquid is viscous, such as that contained in temazepam gel-filled capsules, embolic events can occur, leading to thrombosis and gangrene.

The prescribing doctor must always be aware of the potential harm any prescribed drug can cause, especially if injected. Consider prescribing drug users liquid rather than tablet formulations of 'at-risk' substances such as analgesics and benzodiazepines.

■ Route-specific complications

Injecting drug use carries the greatest risk of infection. Injecting equipment is frequently shared or cursorily cleaned. Dirty and unhygienic injecting habits can result in local or systemic infections and poor injecting technique (particularly femoral injecting) can cause venous or arterial thrombosis. The harm associated with injecting drug use can be reduced by correcting poor injecting technique (*see* box below), providing clean needles and syringes via needle or pharmacy exchange schemes and by giving correct advice on cleaning injecting equipment (*see* box below). Some of the most common harmful practices arise from ignorance, such as injecting towards rather than away from the hand when using the outside of the forearm (therefore against the flow of blood); using contaminated paraphernalia (spoon, filter); and believing only clean needles and syringes are needed to avoid infections.

Safer injecting use

1   Always inject with blood flow.
2   Rotate injecting sites.
3   Use smallest bore needle possible.
4   Avoid neck, breast, feet and hand veins.
5   Mix powders with sterile water and filter solution before injecting.
6   Always dispose of your equipment safely (either in bin provided or by placing your needle inside the syringe and placing both inside drinks can).
7   Avoid injecting into infected areas.
8   Do not inject into swollen limbs even if the veins appear to be distended.
9   Poor veins mean poor technique. Try and see what you are doing wrong.
10 Don't use alone.

Cleaning injecting equipment

To 'bleach clean' injecting equipment you need:

• needle and syringe
• thin undiluted household bleach
• clean cold water
• two clean cups or wide-topped bottles.

Method

1 Pour bleach into one cup (or bottle) and water into another.
2 Draw bleach up with the dirty needle and syringe.
3 Expel bleach in toilet or sink.
4 Repeat steps 2 and 3.
5 Draw water up through needle and syringe.
6 Expel water into toilet or sink.
7 Repeat steps 5 and 6 at least once more, ideally two or three times more.

Points to remember when cleaning equipment

• Boiling plastic syringes melts them.
• Thick bleach is impossible to draw up through a needle.
• Cold water is recommended as warm water may encourage blood to coagulate and hence will be harder to expel through the needle.

Intravenous drug users and their partners should be offered hepatitis A immunisation, hepatitis B testing and immunisation and hepatitis C testing.

■ Safer drug use

Snorting, smoking or swallowing drugs, though safer than injecting, are not routes of ingestion entirely without risk. The simplicity of oral (swallowing, drinking) drug use increases the possibility of experimentation, either through mixing drugs or taking large quantities.

Dangerous drug interactions can occur between drugs that affect the central nervous system such as alcohol, opiates and benzodiazepines. The young naive user in search of the elusive 'high' may be tempted to take a cocktail of drugs. There is particular danger when this cocktail includes opioids such as methadone which, taken alone or in combination with other drugs, can end in death from respiratory depression or aspiration of vomit. All new prescriptions for methadone must be accompanied by a discussion about the danger of overdose and a warning about mixing the drug with alcohol or benzodiazepines.

Prescribing methadone on a blue FP10MDA for daily dispensing and limiting daily dose to no more than 40 mg per day at the beginning of treatment until the tolerance of the user is known are important interventions the GP can make to reduce the potential harm of the drug. However, prescribing of substitution drugs such as methadone and buprenorphine should not be initiated unless the practitioner is trained and experienced in their use. If unsure about prescribing, it is usually better not to intervene but to seek advice from a specialist source. Opiate withdrawals are uncomfortable but they rarely cause death and symptoms such as vomiting and diarrhoea can be alleviated with small doses of appropriate symptomatic medications.

Safer drug use: advice to the non-injector

- Know what you're taking.
- Using cocktails of drugs can be more dangerous than single drug use.
- Use safer route: snorting, smoking or swallowing is usually safer than injecting.
- Look after yourself: eating, sleeping, exercise, rest.

Inhaling drugs is less hazardous than other routes but it is not completely safe. Hot smoke, if not cooled first, can burn the bronchial tissues and inhaled heroin or cocaine can precipitate and worsen asthma. Purified cocaine base (crack cocaine) is usually smoked in a home-made plastic water pipe and produces a sudden intense 'high' comparable to that produced by intravenous use. The effects subside very rapidly and therefore there is a strong tendency for users to repeat the process to regain the 'high'. Inhalations may be repeated as often as every few minutes and can continue for several hours. Overdose of cocaine can result from inhaled use, the physical effects being hypertension and hyperthermia. High doses of cocaine can also precipitate paranoid reactions, as well as heart attacks and strokes, particularly in people with pre-existing cardiac problems.

Substances such as solvents and amyl nitrite do not need to be heated before their psychoactive properties are realised; indeed, their flammability makes applying a flame very dangerous. When inhaling volatile substances it is important that there is an adequate supply of air reaching the lungs along with the vapour. Again, users should be advised not to use alone or in hazardous places such as on roof tops or near river banks.

Snorting of drugs is the least common route of use and is normally associated with powdered cocaine and amphetamine. Prolonged use of these drugs in this way can cause atrophy of the nasal septum and resulting breathing difficulties.

What advice can be given to someone taking a substance of unknown nature and dosage? For some users this uncertainty is part of the 'buzz' of using illicit drugs, though most would like to know what and how much of a drug they are taking. For ecstasy (MDMA) users, some drug outreach services provide health education clinics at rave parties, which can include sample-testing of tablets to confirm they contain MDMA. General practitioners may need to be pragmatic where a young person is experimenting with these drugs. However, it is useful to point out the risks of taking unknown drugs at parties, of mixing drugs and alcohol and of the dangers of 'spiking' drinks. Advice should also be given about the need to keep the body cooled and the need to maintain an adequate intake of water and soft drinks should also be stressed.

The psychotropic effects of some drugs, especially hallucinogenic drugs such as cannabis and LSD, are partly dependent on the expectations and mood of the user and so their use can exacerbate pre-existing anxiety or depression. Again, advice should be given not to use these drugs on one's own.

■ Safer sex

The issue of safer sex can be difficult for doctors or nurses to discuss with their patients. Many professionals feel uncomfortable when talking about sexual issues, especially when it comes to discussing homosexual and non-penetrative methods of sexual activity. Whilst most general practitioners may not be able to discuss in detail the relative risks of the various types of sexual intercourse, they should be able to offer some advice and, where appropriate, direct a patient to another source of information, e.g. Terrence Higgins Trust helpline (0845 1221 200) or their local genitourinary medicine clinic.

Whilst intravenous drug users and their partners are undoubtedly at risk of sexually transmitted diseases such as HIV or hepatitis, they are by no means the only 'at-risk' group. In order to overcome clumsiness in bringing up the issue of safer sex with patients, it should become common practice to discuss these issues with all patients presenting, for example, for contraception advice or travel immunisations. The new patient registration check should include taking a cervical smear history and this is an ideal opportunity to discuss current sexual practice with women. With men, this can also be included, as a routine, when discussing other health promotion issues such as alcohol and smoking.

Where condoms are given, time should be taken to explain their correct use. This should be a practical demonstration using fingers or a plastic model.

Safer sex

- Limit number of sexual partners.
- Ideally be monogamous with current partner.
- Avoid anal intercourse, oral/anal contact and insertion of objects or hand into anus.
- Use condoms for penetrative sex.
- If condom use not possible, consider a diaphragm which offers some protection.
- Remember hepatitis infection can be transmitted through body fluids such as saliva.

The primary care team must be prepared to match the expectations and needs of the patient at the time of presentation, agree on realistic goals and gently facilitate change in behaviour in the direction of safer drug use. Setting unrealistic conditions before helping drug users, for example insisting that they are drug free before providing hepatitis A and B immunisation or hepatitis C testing and treatment, will only result in failure, which is demoralising for doctor and patient alike. Working on other aspects of harm reduction and highlighting a patient's success in reducing harm – such as not sharing needles/syringes or not injecting into thrombosed veins – may help to restore self-esteem and start the process of gaining the patient's trust, as well as bringing about unexpected benefits elsewhere in their lives.

Key points

- All GP practices should be giving advice about reducing harm from drug use, whether or not they provide treatment for drug dependence.
- Small changes in behaviour which reduce harm can have a large health benefit.
- Key areas of advice are about safer ways to use drugs and safer sexual practices.

■ Reference

1 Strang J, Darke S, Hall W *et al.* (1996) Heroin overdose: the case for take-home naloxone. *BMJ.* **312**: 1435.

CHAPTER 10

Drug users with special needs

Drug use and homelessness

Nat Wright

■ The challenges

Homelessness remains a common feature of contemporary UK society. In 2001 in England alone, 184 290 households approaching local authorities were accepted as homeless. The homeless charity Shelter estimated that this represented over 440 000 people. Drug use is the major health concern of single homeless populations.[1] The prevalence of illicit drug use in such UK populations has been described as between 50% and 70%. Approximately 50% also overuse alcohol. Polydrug use, most commonly heroin and crack cocaine, are features of homeless persons' drug use.[2] The combination of unsafe injecting practice and poor personal hygiene means that many homeless drug users have multiple health problems. The chaotic nature of drugs and homelessness also means that other common clinical problems encountered in primary care (for example, diabetes and asthma) are more difficult to manage.

■ Barriers to primary healthcare for homeless drug users

The following have been described as barriers to effective healthcare.[3]

- General practice workload and financial disincentives.
- Limited or poor access to primary care due to opening times, appointment procedures or location.
- GPs feeling they lack the skills to work with homeless drug users.
- Discrimination: notions that some homeless people are deserving of care whereas others are undeserving; belief that homeless people are excessively migrant or mobile;[4] belief that homeless people are violent or antisocial. Some homeless drug users also suffer the triple stigma of drug use, homelessness and discrimination on the grounds of ethnic background.
- Homeless people (particularly rough sleepers) themselves not prioritising their health.

■ Guidelines and policies to help manage clinical risk

Many of the best practice guidelines for drug users are applicable to the homeless drug-using population. They include the following.

- An adequate assessment prior to any prescribing. Though an initial assessment can be ongoing over several consultations, prescribing should not take place until a clear treatment plan has been agreed with the GP, drugs worker and patient.
- Some homeless drug users present to the GP having recently moved into the area. They request the GP to immediately take over the prescription. The GP should only agree to this once the history has been confirmed (usually by telephone or fax correspondence) with the previous prescriber.
- GPs sometimes receive requests from homeless drug users to prescribe medication that is outside current accepted best practice. Such medication includes maintenance benzodiazepines or other opiates (e.g. morphine, dextromoramide, methadone tablets or ampoules). Requests to prescribe such medication should be resisted.
- Due to the multiple morbidity and social difficulties of many homeless drug users, GPs should prescribe only with the support of a drugs worker.
- Encourage the homeless drug user to make appointments rather than 'drop in'. Educate homeless drug users about the appropriate use of emergency appointments, in particular not using such appointments to obtain a repeat sickness certificate.
- Stimulant toxicity (for example, cocaine or amphetamine) sometimes presents in primary care and should be considered a medical emergency.
- Become proficient (and encourage other practice staff to have training) in de-escalation techniques to manage abusive behaviour. It is inaccurate and stigmatising to say that homeless drug users are violent. However, a minority can make inappropriate demands, often when they are new to the service. Explaining practice policies and working procedures can help to minimise the possibility of abusive behaviour.

■ **Effective practice organisation**

■ Specialised versus mainstream general practice

Broadly speaking, there are two primary care models for working with homeless drug users.[5] The first is the mainstream general practice that takes a special interest in working with homeless people. The second is the 'specialised' general practice that works solely with homeless people. The latter has become more common with personal medical services (PMS) legislation. Though some promote the relative merits of one model over the other, it is clear that both models can complement each other.

The merits of the mainstream model are that it integrates and normalises care of homeless drug users into mainstream general practice. The merit of the specialised general practice is that it can provide more focused care. Therefore the strength of the specialised general practice is that it is ideal for providing initial treatment and early rehabilitation for homeless drug users presenting in general practice. Once their acute condition has stabilised and they are familiar with the primary care setting, such patients can be encouraged to register with mainstream general practices. Initially this can require a high degree of support as homeless drug users can become attached to the specialised practice and have difficulty disengaging. This can also be a problem for staff themselves who have been trained in offering continuity of primary care over the long term. However, there is a need for specialised homeless general practices to encourage drug users to register with mainstream general practices at the appropriate time so as to avoid the specialised centre becoming overloaded with patients.

■ Health promotion and homeless people

Promoting health to homeless people is a complex area[6] that is beyond the scope of this chapter. Recent research amongst homeless *Big Issue* vendors highlighted the challenge to deliver health promotion messages to a heterogeneous population of homeless people.[7] It described the need for harm reduction interventions to reduce injecting-related risk behaviour as one priority area. This section seeks to offer practical suggestions as to how such health promotion can take place in the primary care setting.

Preventing complications of intravenous drug use
Offering hepatitis B immunisation is an important part of health promotion to homeless drug users. The sequelae of hepatitis B infection can be devastating. Offering an accelerated schedule (0, 7, 21 days) results in vastly superior completion rates than traditional (0, 1, 6 month) schedules.[8] It is important to remember to give a booster immunisation 12 months after administration of the first dose.

Encouraging homeless drug users to use needle exchange schemes is an important health promotion activity. Needle exchange reduces (but does not eliminate) the prevalence of hepatitis C in the drug-using population, which remains high partly because of the sharing of injecting paraphernalia. Therefore it is important to advise patients not to share filters, spoons, needles or syringes.

Fatal heroin-related overdose is a major cause of death amongst drug users. Primary care staff can help by:

- advising upon not injecting alone
- cautioning against polydrug use or the use of benzodiazepines or alcohol with heroin
- being aware of loss of tolerance after a period of enforced (e.g. prison) or voluntary (including detoxification) abstinence.

It is possible that future developments for homeless people will include programmes for peer administration of naloxone.[9] Certainly previous research has argued that peer involvement of homeless people in health promotion activities will maximise the success of the intervention.

■ Multiagency working

Effective treatment for homeless drug users entails joint working with a wide variety of organisations. The key principles of working with some of the important partners are described below.

Prisons

Many homeless drug users serve custodial sentences. For some it is the only time when they will be abstinent from illicit drugs. Therefore discharge from prison can be a vulnerable time as tolerance can be reduced and the user may restart problematic drug use. General practitioners can help by agreeing to re-register the homeless person after discharge from prison, offering emergency appointments for those discharged from prison on naltrexone medication so as to continue the medication without a break and not restarting pre-prison maintenance opiate medication without reassessment, as reduced tolerance puts the user at risk of opiate overdose.

At the time of writing, the responsibility for much of prison healthcare is being transferred from the Home Office to the NHS. Briefly, for those working in prisons with drug users, this will entail working with primary care organisations (PCOs) which will assume responsibility for prison healthcare. Current areas for future development include:

- if undertaking detoxification in prison, planning detoxification over a reasonable period of time (1–4 weeks dependent upon daily use of heroin) with a reasonable amount of substitute medication to allow adequate control of withdrawal symptoms
- for those admitted on remand or for brief sentencing (less than six weeks), considering continuation of maintenance prescriptions
- working with CARAT teams (counselling, assessment, referral, advice and through care) based within prisons to co-ordinate effective treatment partnerships between primary care and the prisons.

Hospitals

Due to the sequelae of unsafe injecting practice, many homeless drug users are admitted as inpatients on acute hospital wards. The challenges facing the general practitioner when working with hospital colleagues to deliver effective healthcare to homeless drug users include:

- difficulty making a definitive diagnosis and the risk of being discharged from the A and E department without thorough investigation
- hospitals starting patients on a maintenance prescription without any clear plans for continuation of the prescription. A discussion between the hospital and general practitioner prior to starting the prescription can help address this problem
- discharge from hospital with one month's supply of medication such as dihydrocodeine or benzodiazepines but with only one day's supply of methadone. Training of hospital prescribers (particularly junior doctors) in what constitutes an appropriate maintenance prescription can help address the issue of dihydrocodeine and benzodiazepine maintenance scripts being issued for

problematic heroin use. Working with hospital pharmacy departments to dispense a daily pick-up maintenance prescription (either methadone or buprenorphine) of two weeks' duration is clearly an issue for further development and collaboration between primary and secondary care
- patients taking their own discharge to obtain illicit drugs to ameliorate withdrawal symptoms. The primary purpose of prescribing substitute medication to homeless drug users in a hospital setting should be to stabilise the drug problem and so facilitate retention on the ward until the acute physical condition has been successfully treated. Self-discharges are a clinical governance issue as they often take place whilst the user is still suffering serious physical pathology
- difficulty securing adequate follow-up.

Housing departments and social support services

For many GPs their primary point of contact with housing departments is through requests for a letter to support rehousing of homeless individuals. Many GPs receive requests in the consulting room from the homeless person themselves. The GP can save a lot of time by having a practice policy only to provide a supporting letter when requested by the housing department itself.

To help GPs provide a helpful letter, it is important to have some understanding of the concept of 'medical priority' and 'intentionality' as defined in the Homelessness Acts of 1996 and 2002. The 1996 Act placed a statutory responsibility upon city council housing departments to provide housing (or rehousing) for those who are vulnerable as a result of 'old age, mental illness or handicap, physical disability or other special reason'. Such people constituted a medical priority for rehousing and the GP would be approached to provide a letter confirming medical priority. The 2002 Act for England and Wales retains this priority group but it includes the following groups, which could include homeless drug users presenting to their GP.

- People fleeing violence (any type of violence including, but not exclusively, domestic violence).
- People who are vulnerable as a result of spending time in the armed forces or prison or remanded in custody.
- Sixteen and 17 year olds, excluding those whom Social Services are responsible for accommodating.
- Care leavers under the age of 21 who were looked after by Social Services when they were 16 or 17 (with some very limited exceptions).

The Homelessness Act 2002 for Scotland is different in that it aims by 2012 to give every homeless person the right to a home. In effect, this will abolish the concept of 'priority need'. However, throughout the UK, whilst 'medical priority' still places a responsibility upon local authorities, there remains a need for communication between housing departments and general practitioners.

Drug addiction and alcohol addiction are in themselves not considered as medical conditions constituting priority. Therefore a GP letter, whilst making reference to this, should include details of other physical or psychosocial problems that would constitute priority. A brief description of any limitation in their ability to complete simple tasks of daily living will also be of benefit to housing officers. Many housing providers now seek to rehouse homeless people in 'self-contained' accommodation with a support worker to provide 'floating support'. The level of such support can vary depending on the needs of the homeless person. At the time of writing the government has recently introduced a new initiative, 'Supporting People', whereby the rental costs of housing and the support costs (e.g. counselling, meals or other aspects of floating support) will be combined into a single benefit. It is to be hoped that such an initiative will facilitate vulnerable rehoused drug users in maintaining tenancies.

Key points

- Polydrug use and multiple morbidity are common features of homeless persons' drug use.
- Much can be achieved in primary care by mainstream general practice and specialised general practices for homeless people working together.
- Multiagency working with other key stakeholders can optimise health.

■ References

1 Wright N (2002) *Homelessness: a primary care response.* Royal College of General Practitioners, London.
2 Fountain J and Howes S (2002) *Home and Dry? Homelessness and substance use.* Crisis, London.
3 Griffiths S (2002) *Addressing the Health Needs of Rough Sleepers: a paper to the Homelessness Directorate.* Office of the Deputy Prime Minister, London.
4 Tompkins CNE, Wright NMJ, Sheard L *et al.* (2003) Associations between migrancy, health and homelessness: a cross-sectional study. *Health Social Care Commun.* **11**(5): 446–52.
5 Lester H, Wright N and Heath I (2002) Developments in provision of primary health care for homeless people. *Br J Gen Pract.* **52**: 91–2.
6 Power R, French R, Connelly J *et al.* (1999) Health, health promotion and homelessness. *BMJ.* **318**: 590–2.
7 Power R and Hunter G (2001) Developing a strategy for community-based health promotion targeting homeless populations. *Health Educ Res Theory Pract.* **16**(5): 593–602.
8 Wright NMJ, Campbell TL and Tompkins CNE (2002) Comparison of conventional and accelerated hepatitis B immunisation schedules for homeless drug users. *Communicable Dis Public Health.* **5**(4): 324–6.
9 Oldham N and Wright N (2003) A UK policy on 'take home naloxone' for opiate users – strategy or stalemate? *Drugs Educ Prevent Policy.* **10**(2): 105–19.

Women who use drugs

Sue Tyhurst

Women drug users are thought to be under-represented in drug treatment services. This may be because women drug users experience more social and self-directed stigmatisation than do men, especially during pregnancy.[1] Women with children often have fears about their children being taken into care if they disclose their drug use. Women tend to visit their GP more often than men and are usually familiar with this environment. They may prefer to receive treatment for their drug problems in a primary care setting.

Women who do present for help with substance misuse almost always have other problems, which may or may not be contributory factors in their continued drug use. It is important to adopt a holistic approach when helping women drug users, bearing these factors in mind.

■ Housing

Women drug users often live in insecure housing, are vulnerably housed in temporary bed-and-breakfast accommodation or are homeless. Temporary B&B is always mixed gendered so for women fleeing violent relationships this is both unsuitable and often unsafe.

■ Poor physical health

Women may present with a range of health needs resulting from poor nutrition and a chaotic lifestyle as well as harms from the drugs used. They are at risk from sexually transmitted and pelvic inflammatory disease, particularly if supporting their habit by sex work. Women drug users are at higher risk of cervical smear abnormalities and are likely to slip through the cervical screening programme net.

■ Effects on fertility

Periods may be erratic or absent, leading to a belief that there is no need for contraception. However, amenorrhoea should not be assumed to indicate an inability to conceive and advice and availability of effective contraception are essential. Starting treatment with substitute opiates is a time when fertility increases so offering pre-conception counselling or contraceptive advice is especially important at that time.

■ Mental health

Low self-esteem, repetitive unhealthy or abusive relationship patterns, including domestic violence, social isolation and poor self-image or identity are some of the more common issues shared by women drug users. Other less obvious psychiatric conditions may be masked by drug use, commonly depression, anxiety and severe mood swings. These features are especially true of crack cocaine use.

A high percentage of women using substances problematically will have experienced some kind of past trauma, e.g. sexual abuse.[2] This can lead to a range of problems in adulthood stemming from the ensuing damaged internal belief system, such as inability to develop healthy, positive relationships, eating disorders, self-harm, low self-esteem, depression and suicide attempts.

■ Domestic violence

A significant number of drug-using women will be in abusive relationships. A significant number also have male drugs users as partners.[1] Poor self-esteem, lack of confidence and fear mean that women will often remain in abusive and sometimes violent relationships or have a pattern of leaving and returning.

■ Relapse

Giving up drugs can take many attempts, with lapse and relapse a common feature, so it is important not to write women off if they relapse. See the person beyond the stereotype and recognise that building up trust is equally important for you and the patient.

Key points

- Women drug users are less likely to seek treatment and suffer from more stereotyped attitudes than male users.
- Women drug users will often need help with a diversity of social and psychological problems, requiring a co-ordinated and planned approach to treatment across a number of services.
- Prescribing substitute medication is only one facet of treatment. It will have a better chance of success if delivered in conjunction with other social care approaches.

■ References

1 National Treatment Agency (2002) *Models of Care for Treatment of Adult Drug Users.* NTA, London. Available online at: www.nta.nhs.uk

2 Becker J and Duffy C (2002) *Women Drug Users and Drugs Service Provision: service-level responses to engagement and retention.* Briefing Paper 17. Drug Prevention Advisory Service, London.

Caring for the pregnant drug user

Mary Hepburn

Drug-using women, like all women, need appropriate reproductive healthcare to protect and control their fertility and to ensure they have healthy pregnancies if and when they choose.[1,2] Reproductive healthcare for drug-using women should be provided by multidisciplinary teams within services that are easily accessible by any route, including self-referral. The different components of reproductive healthcare should be provided as a continuum either by a single service or by services working in close collaboration to make sure that women do not fall into the gaps that often exist between mainstream services. Primary care offers such continuity and is therefore ideally placed to provide or co-ordinate much of this care.

■ Fertility and general reproductive health

Heroin (and any other drug use that causes a chaotic lifestyle with poor diet and weight loss) can reduce fertility and can cause amenorrhoea. However, the two effects are not always linked so women can be amenorrhoeic but fertile. Any treatment like methadone that stabilises lifestyle and improves general health will increase fertility and this can occur before menstruation resumes. All women attending for drug treatment should therefore be advised about this and, if they do not want to become pregnant, given effective contraception. Long-acting methods such as the progestagen intrauterine system or progestagen implant are especially suitable and can be easily reversed if the woman wants to become pregnant.

To protect both their fertility and any pregnancy they may have, they should be screened for sexually transmitted and other genital tract infections. A cervical smear should be taken if due and rubella status checked. They should be given information about bloodborne virus infections with the offer of screening. Immunisation against hepatitis B (HBV) and hepatitis A (HAV) is worthwhile, the latter especially for women infected with hepatitis C (HCV). They should be given information about the effects of drugs, smoking and alcohol on pregnancy. When they want to conceive it is important that they have a settled lifestyle with their drug use, smoking and alcohol consumption stabilised at the lowest achievable level. Folic acid supplementation should be started in the usual way before contraception is discontinued.

■ Effects of drugs on pregnancy

Drug use is associated with higher rates of mortality and morbidity for mother and baby. However, the drugs commonly used have limited direct effects on pregnancy with most of the adverse effects being due to poor general health and chaotic lifestyle together with other health and social factors common among women from disadvantaged backgrounds.

Long-acting methadone does not carry the increased risk of pre-term labour associated with use of short-acting heroin and there is also considerable evidence of methadone's other medical and social benefits. Available information on the effects of buprenorphine (much of it from illicit use) suggests that dose for dose, it is similar to methadone. While methadone remains the opiate substitute of choice, women stabilised on buprenorphine at the time of conception can be maintained on this during pregnancy. All opiates can cause withdrawal symptoms in the baby. Those due to dihydrocodeine can be especially severe but otherwise there seems to be little difference in severity although those due to methadone are later in onset and more prolonged.

Benzodiazepines increase the risk of cleft palate but the risk to the individual fetus is still small. They also cause neonatal withdrawals that are especially severe, often prolonged and are less easily treated than those due to opiates. Withdrawals due to combined opiate and benzodiazepine use are disproportionately severe and difficult to treat. No other drug causes significant neonatal withdrawals although alcohol and tobacco can cause mild withdrawals that do not need treatment.

Cocaine use can cause placental separation and pre-term rupture of membranes with many other effects variously reported. However, adverse effects seem largely confined to heavy chaotic use of cocaine, especially crack cocaine. Alcohol causes reduced fetal growth and, rarely in the UK, the combination of effects known as fetal alcohol syndrome.

■ Management of pregnant drug-using women

Care should be provided by a multidisciplinary team. Early stabilisation of drug use is important. Detoxification from opiates is safe at any speed and any stage of pregnancy but should only be undertaken if appropriate. Detoxification from benzodiazepines is safe for the fetus but cover with a short reducing course of diazepam is advisable to prevent maternal convulsions. While this may not achieve long-lasting abstinence, it should be encouraged in order to reduce exposure of the fetus and can be repeated if necessary. Women using methadone as well as benzodiazepines should reduce and if possible discontinue the latter first and the dose of methadone may need to be increased to help them do so. There is no evidence to support maintenance therapy for any other type of drug apart from opiates. While stabilisation at the lowest comfortable dose is the objective, external factors may influence stability and the dose may need to be varied accordingly (up or down) throughout pregnancy. Pregnant drug-using women should be offered screening for HIV, HBV and HCV and for those not immune (especially those who are HCV PCR+ve) pregnancy can be a good time to administer immunisation against HAV and HBV.

A detailed scan at 18–20 weeks is justified for women using benzodiazepines but maternity care should otherwise be according to individual circumstances. Additional monitoring of the fetus is only indicated if there are clinical concerns but it is important to remember that these women have potentially high-risk pregnancies. They are therefore not suitable for midwife-only care although much of their care can be delivered by midwives. General medical and social problems should be addressed. A multidisciplinary meeting at 32 weeks' gestation allows identification of problems, setting of goals and planning of management.

The vulnerable babies of drug-using women will especially benefit from breastfeeding, which will also reduce the severity of neonatal drug withdrawals. All drug-using women (except those who are HIV+ve) should be encouraged to breastfeed regardless of drugs used, dose or pattern of use. Breastfeeding is not contraindicated for women who are HCV PCR+ve.

Effective contraception should be provided in the immediate postpartum period and both the progestagen implant and intrauterine system can be fitted before postnatal discharge.

Social support should include support with parenting and be continued after postnatal discharge. However, there should be a clear distinction between family support and child protection, with the latter separately addressed only if necessary.

Key points

- Drug-using women need comprehensive reproductive healthcare provided as a continuum to protect and control their fertility.
- If provided with appropriate services, drug-using women attend regularly for care and can have healthy pregnancies at times of their choosing.

■ References

1 Scottish Executive (2003) *Getting Our Priorities Right: good practice guidance for working with children and families affected by substance misuse.* Scottish Executive, Edinburgh.
2 Advisory Council on the Misuse of Drugs (2003) *Hidden Harm: responding to the needs of children of problem drug users.* Home Office, London.

Parents who misuse drugs

Jane Powell

An increasing population of problem drug users are becoming parents and increasing numbers of young children are growing up in households where parental drug use is a feature of their lives. A recently published report, *Hidden Harm*,[1] estimates that there are between 200 000 and 300 000 children in England and Wales where one or both parents have serious drug problems. This represents about 2–3% of children under 16. Most parents who use drugs genuinely want to do what is best for their children and many will never come to the attention of Social Services or other agencies despite the potential risks to the health, development and safety of their children. These effects can be seen at every stage of their lives from conception onwards.

■ What are the risks to children?

Parents who misuse drugs are more likely to be economically deprived, to be unemployed, to live in temporary accommodation and have previous contact with the criminal justice system. They also often have a greater range of personal difficulties than parents who do not use drugs, with a particularly strong association with domestic violence and mental health problems.

In these circumstances children can be highly vulnerable; whilst there should be no automatic presumption of neglect or abuse it is reasonable that parenting ability should be assessed. Drug use can affect parenting capacity directly through the effects on the parents' mental state and ability to make judgements and indirectly because of a possible chaotic lifestyle and impoverished home environment. A level of physical neglect is very likely in households where resources are diverted to funding and using drugs. If a parent's main attachment is to a drug there will be implications for their attachment to their children.

■ Current national guidance

The Department of Health, with other government departments, has recently published the *Framework for the Assessment of Children in Need and Their Families*.[2] The guidance sets out a clear expectation that all professionals working with children and families will contribute to the ongoing assessment of, and provision of services to, children in need. This requirement specifically extends to professionals whose main focus of work is with adults; for example, workers in substance misuse services. The framework stresses interagency collaboration as one of the keys to successfully improving outcomes for children, with health professionals playing a particularly important role.

The Standing Conference on Drug Abuse has published policy guidelines on working with parents who are problem drug users, including pregnant women.[3] These guidelines recommend the development of local policies involving drug services, maternity services, paediatricians, GPs and Social Services.

■ The role of GPs and other health professionals

It is important that professionals should be aware of their own views and prejudices. Drug users can evoke strong feelings and can be easily stereotyped. It is the parental behaviour (for example, intoxication, leaving children unattended, dangerously poor supervision, physical or emotional abuse or neglect) that represents the risk to the child and not the label of heroin or crack user. Nor should parents who become abstinent necessarily be assumed to have become better or safer parents in the absence of other evidence. Withdrawal from drugs can significantly impair the capacity to tolerate stress and anxiety.

Health professionals have a responsibility to refer concerns to key agencies involved, usually Social Services. Families must always be told about the referral and the reason for it. The issue of confidentiality may compound difficulties and professionals may feel unsure about their responsibilities in this respect. *Working Together to Safeguard Children*[4] and *The Framework for the Assessment of Children in Need and Their Families*[2] state very clearly that where there are concerns about the welfare of a child these concerns over-ride the right of an adult to confidentiality. Unlike alcohol use, drug use is illegal. It is expensive and usually takes place in private. Guilt, denial, fear and suspicion of all professionals can mean that parents who use drugs are very difficult to engage.

Fearful that a referral to Social Services will trigger the automatic removal of their children, parents may often set themselves the unrealistic goal of rapid detoxification and abstinence where stabilisation and maintenance would be more realistic. Where parents have themselves experienced a troubled background, they may hope that children will 'make up' for their past problems and give them a reason to be drug free. This may lead to attempts to detoxify too rapidly with the risk of relapse.

Multiagency work is not easy and not self-evidently useful at times; some professionals may have had experiences of poor responses from referrals to Social Services, ranging from punitive or ill judged to a disregarding of concerns expressed. Clarity of roles, responsibilities and expectations can improve working relationships as can the use of written policies and protocols.

Key points

- Drug use is not a single phenomenon. It encompasses a wide range of behaviours some of which are incompatible with good parenting. It is important that professionals look at people's behaviour and not just at the label attached to them.
- A sensitive and helpful response by professionals should include an acknowledgement of the adult's strengths as a parent and an understanding of the dilemmas faced.
- Treatment or control of drug use, rather than enforced and unsuccessful abstinence, will provide stability for many parents and their children.
- Most parents want what is best for their children. Parents who use drugs are usually aware of the adverse impact on their parenting role. Many can be successfully engaged in treatment and contact with other agencies.

■ References

1 Home Office (2003) *Hidden Harm. Responding to the needs of children of problem drug users*. Stationery Office, London.
2 Departments of Health, Home Office, Education and Employment (2000) *Framework for the Assessment of Children in Need and Their Families*. Stationery Office, London.
3 Local Government Drugs Forum and Standing Conference on Drug Abuse (1997) *Drug Using Parents: policy guidelines for inter-agency working*. Stationery Office, London.
4 Departments of Health, Home Office, Education and Employment (1999) *Working Together to Safeguard Children*. Stationery Office, London.

Black and minority ethnic (BME) drug use

Dima Abdulrahim

■ Prevalence and patterns of drug use

Prevalence rates of drug use among BME populations are lower than those of the majority white population; low levels are particularly evident among south Asians and black Africans. Although overall levels of drug use are similar among black Caribbeans and whites, this is largely because of the high use of cannabis in the former group.[1]

However, drug use amongst BME populations is significant and is increasing. Moreover, a combination of factors that characterise the lives of many BME people, in particular risk factors that revolve around social exclusion and deprivation, means that the context within which drug use exists provides an environment in which it can be particularly problematic.[2]

Studies suggest that, overall, BME populations use a similar range of substances to their white peers. There are, however, different patterns and levels of problematic drug use amongst the different groups. African Caribbeans are more likely than all other groups to present to services for a primary crack cocaine problem and problematic use may also focus on cannabis. This does not mean that these communities are not affected by heroin; individuals do present to services for opiate users and, whilst smoking is more common, injecting does occur. Heroin use often starts in prison or is started to manage the comedown from crack.

Heroin is often the drug of choice of south Asian populations, who are more likely to smoke than inject. However, there is some evidence of injecting and anecdotal evidence of an increase in injecting, especially amongst young people. The low uptake of needle exchange facilities is cause for concern, as is possible lack of knowledge about transmission of bloodborne infections.[3] Little is known about drug use among newly arriving communities, including refugees and asylum seekers. The use of khat is restricted to Somalis and some problematic use has been noted. Heroin use has been noted amongst Vietnamese and Turkish-speaking communities.

■ Uptake of treatment

There is strong evidence that BME drug users – and south Asians in particular – are under-represented in treatment services throughout the country. This may not be so much the case in London but even in the capital, whilst African Caribbean and Indian drug users are utilising drug services, black Africans, Pakistanis and Bangladeshis are under-represented, as are drug users from more recently established communities. There is also plenty of anecdotal evidence that services are often not able to retain BME users in treatment. However, where there is concerted effort to work with these groups, good retention rates can be achieved.[4]

Evidence about how BME patients perceive the accessibility of drug treatment within primary care is contradictory. Some studies show that south Asian and other BME drug users would be more likely to approach a GP than a drug service and commentators have recommended the development of such services.[5,6] Another study showed that on the contrary, BME users – and south Asians in particular – were less likely to see their GP about their drug use than their white peers and in some instances the differences were striking.[3]

■ Barriers to uptake of treatment

Studies have identified a number of barriers to the uptake of drug treatment in all settings.

1 Denial that drug use exists in some communities (e.g. south Asian) by communities and professionals alike.
2 Fear of breach of confidentiality.
3 Ethnicity of staff.
4 Lack of understanding of BME cultures.[3]
5 Lack of appropriate service responses in terms of:

- underdevelopment of treatment for crack cocaine[4]
- paucity of response to cannabis
- opiate focus of drug treatment, especially by community services
- harm reduction focus on injecting; needs of non-injectors are often marginalised
- residential rehabilitation services have been analysed as least capable of meeting the needs of diverse populations.[3]

Key points

- Drug use prevalence rates amongst black and minority ethnic populations are lower than in the general population but are nonetheless significant, increasing and exist in a high-risk context of social exclusion.
- Issues to be considered include cannabis use, a response to crack use and poor knowledge of transmission of bloodborne infections.
- GPs are in a unique position to work with BME users as they often have substantial experience of dealing with the needs of culturally and socially diverse populations.

■ References

1 Ramsey M, Baker P, Goulden C *et al.* (2001) *Drug Misuse Declared in 2000: results from the British Crime Survey.* Home Office Research, Development and Statistics Directorate, London.
2 Fountain J, Bashford J, Winters M *et al.* (2003) *Black and Minority Ethnic Communities in England: a review of the literature on drug use and related service provision.* National Treatment Agency, London.
3 Sangster D, Shiner M, Patel K *et al.* (2002) *Delivering Drug Services to Black and Minority Ethnic Communities.* Drug Prevention Advisory Service, London.
4 Harocopos A, Dezlee D, Turnball P *et al.* (2003) *On the Rocks: a follow-up study of crack users in London.* City Roads, South Bank University, National Treatment Agency, London.
5 Johnson MRD and Carroll M (1995) *Dealing with Diversity: good practice in drug prevention work with racially and culturally diverse communities.* Home Office, London.
6 Chaudry MA, Sherlock K and Patel K (1997) *Drugs and Ethnic Health Project: Oldham and Tameside.* University of Central Lancashire, Preston.

■ Useful contacts

Commission for Racial Equality (CRE)
St Dunstan's House
201–211 Borough High Street
London SE1 1GZ
www.cre.gov.uk

UCLAN – Centre for Ethnicity and Health
Harrington Building
Faculty of Health
University of Central Lancashire
Preston PR1 2HE
www.uclan.ac.uk

Young people and drugs

Tom Aldridge

Substance use and misuse by young people (defined as those under the age of 18) is a cause for concern, although the British Crime Surveys[1] suggest that Class A drug use by young people stabilised in the 1990s after a rise in the previous decade. However, this masks statistically significant increases in the use of cocaine and ecstasy but reductions in the use of LSD, magic mushrooms and amphetamines. Prevalence is higher amongst vulnerable groups, such as young offenders, school excludees and truants, and 'looked-after' children. Alcohol, tobacco smoking, cannabis use and volatile substance misuse are also issues that need to be addressed.[2]

Statistics published in 2003 suggest that among 11–15 year olds in England, prevalence of drug use in 2002 was 20%, with 11% taking drugs in the last month. The prevalence of drug use increased sharply with age: only 6% of 11 year olds had used drugs in the last year compared to 36% of 15 year olds. Cannabis was the most frequently reported illicit drug used in the last year (13%). One percent had used heroin and 1% had used cocaine in the last year.[3]

Young people may experience physical or mental health problems as a result of drug use. Drug use may also lead to related lifestyle problems involving changes in friendships and family relationships, poor school, college or work performance, financial problems, criminal behaviour and associations, getting in trouble with the police and conflict with parents/carers. Young people's drug use creates problems for families and the wider community but some of these problems may partly be due to adults' and society's response to young people's drug use rather than the drug itself.

Young people may also be adversely affected because of the use of drugs by others around them, especially parents/carers, brothers and sisters, other family members and their friends. The government estimates that there are between 200 000 and 300 000 children of problem drug users in England and Wales.[4]

'Risks' and 'problems' may be perceived very differently by young people and adults. Young people sometimes see risk as attractive. Adults are often very selective about their perceptions of risk and encourage young people to be involved in certain risky activities such as outdoor pursuits. Young people may also not see drug-related problems as being of much significance or may enjoy status and attention from experiencing them. Parents or teachers may see any contact with drugs as a problem whilst the young person concerned may see their drug use as a pleasure.

When considering drug problems with young people, it is important to assess risk realistically and when there are problems, to find out what exactly they are, who they are a problem for and how the young person involved feels about them.

■ Services for young drug users

Services for young people are an important strand in the government's Updated Drug Strategy.[5] As a consequence, there is some provision of dedicated counselling, assessment and harm reduction services for young drug users in 70% of local authority areas.[6] There are also arrangements for funding and access to detoxification and residential services although these may not necessarily be provided locally.

These services are specifically for young drug users and for parents who are concerned about their children's use. They are therefore organised differently from traditional adult services and may be integrated within community and adolescent mental health services or generic youth counselling and advice services.

■ The role of general practice

Because many young people and their families already know and use their GP service, the primary care team can play an important role in responding to drug problems amongst the younger age group. This might include:

- providing accurate information about help with substance misuse that is available from local services or national organisations. This can include provision of leaflets and poster displays
- sensitively exploring issues around possible drug and alcohol use when young people consult for other reasons
- counselling young users and family members about the effects of drugs and alcohol and how to reduce harm from their use
- helping young drug users to optimise their physical health by monitoring and giving advice about weight, nutrition, sexual health and bloodborne viruses
- working in partnership with the local young people's service to meet young people's needs arising from substance misuse
- referral on to dedicated drug services when appropriate.

Prescribed medication has a minimal role. There are no drugs licensed for the treatment of addictions for young people under 18 nor is there any evidence base for the effectiveness of antagonist or substitute treatment programmes in this age group. Work with younger drug users and parents extends beyond a 'medical model'. In particular, young people and parents will need to feel that GPs and practice staff are approachable, non-judgemental, non-patronising and knowledgeable. Confidentiality will be particularly important to young people. Parents will often need reassurance and support in understanding and realistically helping their children.

Key points

- Substance use by young people is common but not always problematic.
- Young people need a different type of service from adults and these services are now being developed as a priority.
- GPs can offer information, advice and support to young users and their families.

■ References

1 Home Office Research Findings (1994, 1996, 1998, 2000, 2001–02) *Prevalence of Drug Use: key findings from the British Crime Survey.* Research, Development and Statistics Directorate, Home Office, London.
2 Health Advisory Service (2001) *The Substance of Young Needs.* Health Advisory Service, London.
3 Home Office Statistical Bulletin (2003) *Statistics on Young People and Drug Misuse: England 2002.* Home Office, London.
4 Advisory Council on Misuse of Drugs (2003) *Hidden Harm. Responding to the needs of children of problem drug users.* Stationery Office, London.
5 Strategy Directorate (2002) *Updated Drug Strategy 2002.* Home Office, London.
6 National Treatment Agency (2003) *Annual Report 2002/03.* NTA, London.

■ Useful contacts

www.dailydose.net
Updated weekly, provides latest details on patterns of drug use.

www.cascade-drugs.org.uk
Drug information service for young people and parents. Includes drug facts, discussion boards and a problem page for parents.

www.talktofrank.com
Information about the effects of drugs and how to find local services for young people. Can also phone the National Drugs Helpline (FRANK) on 0800 77 66 00.

CHAPTER 11

What do drug users need from the general practitioner?

Alan Joyce

No one individual can claim to know what drug users want. To claim to have the answer to this question would be presumptuous indeed and would perpetuate the idea that drug users are a homogeneous group with identical problems, needs and expectations of what they want from their GP. I am writing this chapter based on my own experience as a user in treatment and my work as a user advocate working with the Alliance (formerly known as the Methadone Alliance). For these reasons the term 'drug user' should be taken to refer to opiate users in this chapter.

The evidence base about what users want is poor and reflects the fact that users, historically, have been seen as the recipients of treatment rather than as informed consumers of care who are capable of determining with a supportive GP the kind of care that best meets their needs.

While musing on the question 'What do drug users want?', my first temptation was to give a seemingly obvious answer – a script or perhaps a more sophisticated variant of the same, such as diamorphine on demand. Yet is a script all that drug users really want or need from a GP? The longer I mused on such a simple reply, the less appropriate it seemed. Perhaps one may arrive at a more appropriate response by considering the whole range of health and social problems that drug users experience. These are well documented in preceding chapters and include sepsis, bloodborne virus infections, high rates of smoking and alcohol consumption, poor diets, mental health difficulties and health problems associated with social exclusion, poor housing and poverty.

In many respects these needs are not so different from the problems non-drug using patients would reasonably expect their general practitioner to recognise and deal with. Many of them can be and are managed very effectively within general practice although some may require onward referral to a specialist. Why then do we receive consistent anecdotal reports of drug users being refused general medical care?

Unfortunately there is very little hard evidence to show the extent to which the denial of general medical care to drug users is a problem. A recent small-scale survey of GPs' attitudes to drug users conducted by the Gwent Users Alliance was illuminating. Seventy questionnaires were sent out to GPs in the

South Wales area. Six of the 30 GPs who responded stated that they would be unwilling to provide general medical care to drug users. Even though this was just one small study, it is suggestive of a problem that needs to be addressed.

Denial of general medical care to a drug user would appear to set such GPs at odds with the following guidelines:

> Drug misusers have the same entitlement as other patients to the services provided by the National Health Service. It is the responsibility of *all doctors* (my emphasis) to provide care for both the general health needs and drug-related problems, whether or not the patient is ready to withdraw from drugs.[1]

The General Medical Council is equally clear on this issue:

> No-one should be discriminated against because of their ability to pay, their social position, their health status, their race, religion, sex, lifestyle or their age. Indeed, those whose needs are greatest, for whatever reason, even if their illnesses are to some extent self-inflicted, have the same rights as anyone else and if equity is to be respected they may well require a greater share of the available resources to maintain life or restore health.[2]

■ Difficulties in accessing GP care

Even if a GP is ostensibly prepared to register drug users, it can be difficult to access GP care for a variety of reasons. Some of the barriers to access may be subtle and unintentional.

The first hurdle can be trying to register with a GP in the first place. Some users may not understand or lack information about the registration process. Users moving area, which many do as part of an attempt at change, can find this a particular problem. Knowledge of the healthcare system and how to access it can be poor and the requisite information difficult to access. There are additional problems for the more marginalised or chaotic user who may be homeless, living in squats or hostel accommodation and have poor literacy skills.

Stepping into a surgery for the first time can be difficult and intimidating if the attitude of a practice to drug users is unknown beforehand. Fear of rejection is itself a deterrent against engagement. In many practices the clock appears not to have moved since I was first escorted to the surgery door in Hampstead in 1980. Many users who have had similar experiences of stigmatisation and discrimination in the NHS in the past will be reluctant to risk subjecting themselves to it again. Users are not isolated individuals. They meet and share experiences, knowledge and information. The negative experiences of users are relayed to others, become received wisdom and serve to discourage other users from engagement with general practice.

Having built up the courage and crossed the practice threshold, the next hurdle to be negotiated is the attitude and training of staff working in the practice. They can be instrumental in encouraging or discouraging the user from seeking care. Receptionists can perceive their role to be that of protecting the practice, the doctor and 'proper' patients from potentially difficult clients. They may profess an ability to 'detect a drug user from a mile off' (an expression I have heard more than once). Is it the dog on a string that gives us away, our bedraggled clothing, body odour (junkies are notorious soap dodgers) or our furtive shifty appearance? More often than not judgements will be made on the basis of appearance, received wisdom, stereotypes or projection of personal beliefs and experience of reception staff. This can lead to subtle, sometimes unconscious discrimination. From a disapproving look to shouting confidential details across a crowded reception area, the user can easily be made to feel unwelcome.

■ Difficulties in accessing treatment for drug dependency

A look at the problems facing a user seeking treatment specific for their opiate dependence brings me to what I call the 'Oliver Twist' moment or the 'Please sir, can I have some more?' experience. Actually, in many cases this is not so much 'more' as 'Please sir, can I have anything?'.

One patient illustrates the difficulties users can face. Jill had managed to negotiate the barriers discouraging engagement and made a point, based on prior experience, of building a relationship of trust with her GP prior to making any request for treatment specific to her opiate dependence. Jill was approaching 60 years of age, had been with the practice for some time and had been open about her opiate dependence. She was also suffering from hepatitis C and chest and heart problems, including endocarditis, for which she was receiving treatment.

She finally built up the confidence to enable her to risk the 'Oliver' question. She had been on methadone maintenance treatment for several years in her previous practice until the retirement of her GP. Her notes would have shown that she responded positively to this and had been an exemplary patient. Her request for a methadone maintenance prescription was met with the following response from this GP: 'You are a social evil, there is the door, use it'.

She was precipitated into depression and crisis by this response to her desperate plea for help, a plea for help that took time, trust and courage to make. She left the practice but was lucky enough to receive help from the Methadone Alliance and secure the treatment she needed elsewhere. Why was she denied a treatment that had evidently served her well in the past?

■ Reasons why GPs may not treat opiate dependence

It is important to acknowledge that GPs can and do have legitimate anxieties about engaging with drug users and providing treatment specific to their condition. However, there is also a deeply embedded culture within elements of the profession whereby received wisdom, prejudice, moral judgements and personal beliefs continue to be represented and legitimised as clinical judgement. Left unchallenged, such judgement may be actively deployed to deny patients access to evidence-based treatment of proven effectiveness.

■ Training

The lack of appropriate training at all stages prior to accreditation as a GP is significant. Training in the management of substance misuse may be as little as four hours in total before becoming a GP. It is understandable that GPs identify this as a reason why they feel reluctant to engage with users. The recent growth in training opportunities should now enable any GP to acquire the knowledge and skills they need.

■ Not enough time

Given the average GP's workload, this is an understandable excuse but if it were a valid one for refusing treatment, one could anticipate that other patient groups would be equally likely to have treatment denied for this reason. The objection is predicated on an assumption that all drug users require the same treatment for their drug use and that any such treatment will be time consuming. While it is certainly true that some drug users present with complex needs and problems, it is equally true that many users do not. Some may require far less support than patients with other chronic relapsing medical conditions who are routinely treated within general practice. All that may be needed for the long-term stable maintained user is a monthly appointment for a little TLC and a methadone script.

■ Opiate dependency is a self-inflicted, social problem

Heart disease, obesity, smoking-related illness, late-onset diabetes and a host of other morbidities can be described as lifestyle-related and thereby self-inflicted conditions. The objection that doctors are being asked to treat a social problem rather than a clinical condition is one that is often heard in relation to drug users. Interestingly, the police have been known to argue the opposite, that they are being asked to police and imprison people suffering from a medical condition.

These objections are addressed explicitly by the GMC.

> The investigations or treatment you provide or arrange must be based on your clinical judgement of patients' needs and the likely effectiveness of the treatment. You must not allow your views about a patient's lifestyle, culture, beliefs, race, gender, sexuality, disability, age or social or economic status, to prejudice the treatment you provide or arrange. You must not refuse or delay treatment because you believe that patients' actions have contributed to their condition.[3]

■ Fear of overwhelming numbers

This fear of being swamped by drug users seeking treatment is difficult to justify or accept. It may be based on the unfortunate experience of a small number of GPs. One could criticise it as a self-fulfilling prophecy. By denying treatment to drug users for this reason, a scarcity of treatment is created and users seeking treatment will gravitate to practices they know will provide it. This should be seen not so much as a reason for denying care but rather as a compelling indicator of the need for greater provision of this kind of treatment. The situation is not helped by the failure of many other drug treatment services to meet demand.

There is also a worrying subtext. This language is associated with prejudice and discrimination. Fear of 'overwhelming numbers' is highly inflammatory in certain circumstances and has a history of being deployed to justify discrimination against minority groups. Any practitioners working in Southall, Leicester or Brick Lane using this phrase to justify limiting the numbers of Asian patients in their practice would find the charge of discrimination rightly raised.

■ Wary of harm reduction and uncertain over the aims of treatment

As indicated before, this is a legacy of inadequate training. Support and guidance are also available from drugs workers and shared-care schemes.

■ Drug users seen as demanding, devious and violent

This may reflect the personal experience of a small number of GPs who have encountered difficulties treating drug-using patients. Received wisdom becomes accepted 'lore' and then established 'knowledge'. Once accepted as such, it in turn informs and legitimises practice and in this case can serve to justify denial of treatment and care.

Drug users are human beings and as such can be expected to embody the behavioural traits and characteristics of our species. Undoubtedly, a small number of drug users may be difficult, have behavioural problems and be demanding or even aggressive and violent. However, this could probably be said of other patient groups: not all 18-year-old working-class youths are knife-wielding thugs, not all members of the black community are ganja-smoking 'dreads', nor are all inner-city unemployed kids muggers.

Drug users, as with any other disparate group of people with one problem, background or condition in common, are individuals and best treated as such. Treating a stereotype is unlikely to produce positive results, treating an individual will.

■ Need for resources and payment to acknowledge the extra work

While there are many, including myself, who believe that treatment of drug use should have been included as a core service under the new GP Contract, providing a treatment service to drug users will now be remunerated as a National Enhanced Service. It's official! GPs can no longer shelter behind the myth that good-quality care of drug users is exclusively the domain of specialist treatment centres and has no place in primary care.

■ Drug users are individual human beings

Good Medical Practice[3] says it all.

> Patients must be able to trust doctors with their lives and well-being. To justify that trust, we as a profession have a duty to maintain a good standard of practice and care and to show respect for human life. In particular as a doctor you must:
>
> - make the care of your patient your first concern
> - treat every patient politely and considerately
> - respect patients' dignity and privacy
> - listen to patients and respect their views
> - give patients information in a way they can understand
> - respect the rights of patients to be fully involved in decisions about their care
> - keep your professional knowledge and skills up to date
> - recognise the limits of your professional competence
> - be honest and trustworthy
> - respect and protect confidential information
> - make sure that your personal beliefs do not prejudice your patients' care
> - act quickly to protect patients from risk if you have good reason to believe that you or a colleague may not be fit to practise
> - avoid abusing your position as a doctor
> - work with colleagues in the ways that best serve patients' interests.
>
> In all these matters you must never discriminate unfairly against your patients or colleagues. And you must always be prepared to justify your actions to them.

Drug users want just what any other patient would from their GPs – good-quality general healthcare and non-judgemental, evidence-led treatment for their specific chronic medical condition. Above all, I would suggest that drug users need and want to be treated with empathy. Any GP who is able to set out on a path that is illuminated by this beacon will be on the path to a positive and rewarding treatment outcome for both themselves and their drug-using patient.

Key points

- Drug users are human beings and individuals who deserve the same courtesy, respect and dignity as any other patient presenting for care.
- No GP should deny a drug user general medical care.
- GPs can play a key role in a drug user's health, minimisation of harm and recovery. Stability on long-term maintenance prescribing is a valid form of recovery in and of itself.
- A warm and welcoming practice can make all the difference between a user presenting and staying in treatment or not.
- Empathy and trust are valued by users and will be reciprocated.
- Treating and working with drug users can be an enriching and rewarding process for doctor and patient.

■ References

1 Department of Health, Scottish Office Department of Health, Welsh Office, Department of Health and Social Services, Northern Ireland (1999) *Drug Misuse and Dependence – guidelines on clinical management*. Stationery Office, London.
2 General Medical Council (2000) *Guidance on Good Practice: priorities and choices*. General Medical Council, London.
3 General Medical Council (2001) *Good Medical Practice*. General Medical Council, London.

■ Useful contacts

The Methadone Alliance (The Alliance)
A unique national user-led charity providing advocacy, helpline support, training, service user group development and other services to drug users seeking, or having problems with, treatment for their drug use. The Alliance also provides expertise, support, training and other services to the NTA, DATs, treatment services and other professional bodies involved in drug treatment and related fields. The Alliance service is open to all drug users who are experiencing problems, irrespective of drug/drugs used, but still retains a core focus on the problems of opiate and opiate-dependent polydrug users.
Helpline: 0208 374 4395
Email: methadone.alliance@blueyonder.co.uk
www.m-alliance.org.uk

UK Harm Reduction Alliance
An alliance of users, professionals, drug workers, researchers and others dedicated to promoting harm reduction-based approaches to drug use and treatment in the UK. The discussion lists are highly recommended.
UKHRA-Discussion – diverse membership of supporters of harm reduction.
UKHRA-Users – primarily for drug users and activists but has a small number of nominated professionals among its contributors.
www.ukhra.org

Addiction Treatment Forum online
An excellent source of facts and information as well as up-to-date research findings. Highly recommended.
www.atforum.com/

Danish Drug Users Union
One of the first and one of the best.
www.brugerforeningen.dk/bfny.nsf/pagesuk/UKMP6.html?OpenDocument

National Drug Users Development Agency
1st floor, 388 Old Street
London EC1V 9CT
NDUDA represents the interests of drug users to government and professionals in the drugs field. It supports the development and networking of drug users' groups.
Telephone: 0207 739 6633

CHAPTER 12

Families and carers

Vivienne Evans

This chapter discusses the role families play in supporting and caring for problematic drug users. It emphasises the need to recognise the importance of the role of families and that families need support in their own right, not just as the carer of the user. Despite a body of evidence on the impact of alcohol misuse on the family, research into the impact of illicit drug misuse is limited.

The term 'family' means any person in a close and supportive relationship with a drug user.

There is growing concern about the needs of families affected by drug use and the best way of meeting those needs. There is an increasing recognition that drug misuse affects the entire family and the communities in which these families live. The needs of these families, however, are not well known or documented. Despite research which indicates that engaging families improves treatment outcomes, arrests declining family health and improves the impact of drugs education,[1] families in England affected by problems with drugs continue to be at best condescended to or, at worst, actively excluded. Shame, guilt and isolation are common experiences, matched with a constant struggle with the daily trauma of problematic drug use.

■ The impact of problematic drug use on families

It is well established that living in close contact with someone with a drug problem leads to a high level of physical and psychological stress. Short-term negative effects include feeling angry, lonely, isolated, tired, drained, unsupported, anxious, depressed, suicidal, guilty, tearful, apprehensive, worried, fearful, tense and confused.[2]

Families respond to drug use in different ways.

- *Denial*: long-term denial, rather than facing up to issues, can result in greater anxiety and conflict.
- *Self blame*: families often blame themselves, particularly for a child's drug use. This is reinforced if treatment agencies regard the family as the cause or part of the problem and this can be a significant barrier to accessing support.
- *Blame*: in this case the family assigns responsibility for the problem to others,

for example, social workers, drugs agencies or the NHS. This results in anger towards agencies and makes it difficult for support to be accessed and developed.

- *'Tough love'*: families can respond by creating a physical or emotional distance between themselves and the user, sometimes resulting in removing the user from the family home.

Longer term effects include changes in physical health such as shingles, ulcers, raised blood pressure and/or psychological health, including anorexia, depression, panic attacks and 'nervous breakdown'. Family members also report the effects of the drug user's behaviour on their own behaviour, including increases in their own drug, tobacco and alcohol use and eating disorders.[2]

One indicator of physical and psychological stress is the number of times family members visit a primary care setting. One study in Canada revealed that families living with an addiction problem visited their doctor frequently with a number of symptoms, both psychological and physical, that are usually associated with living with chronic and ongoing stress.[3]

Family life is also subject to social disruption.

- *Rituals*: family rituals which serve to unite and reunite families are seriously affected by problematic drug behaviour.
- *Routines*: are disrupted; for example, children are not picked up from school and mealtimes tend to lack consistency, if they happen at all.
- *Roles*: family members tend to compensate for the drug user by accommodating his or her role and function in the family; for example, children become their parents' carers.
- *Communication*: families either try to avoid the problem and not talk about it or do talk about it and increase the emotional content of communication which leads to conflict and further anxiety.
- *Social life*: young people tend not to bring friends home because they are worried about disclosure; families often report feeling alienated from friends and communities and fear they are the topic of gossip; many family members feel they cannot leave the drug user alone at home and have little energy to go out.
- *Finances*: difficulties often arise both as a direct result of the drug user's behaviour and through families' attempts to help by actually purchasing the necessary drugs or by repaying debts; drug users steal from their families; families pay for rehabilitation treatment. Grandparents who care for grandchildren experience problems arising from child benefit books being held by loan sharks to cover debts incurred by the user; grandparents are not able to claim child benefit unless the parent agrees to this.
- *Employment*: financial difficulties are exacerbated in some families because a family member gives up work, either because they are caring for the user or because they cannot cope with the twin demands of home and work.

The impact of problem drug use on children is a matter of particular, and increasing, concern. In addition to the disruptions described above, these children are exposed to:

- actual drug use by parents and others, and safety hazards if, for example, needles are left around at home
- criminality
- domestic violence
- verbal and emotional abuse, particularly when the parent is craving or withdrawing
- educational disruption and underachievement
- feelings of hurt, shame, rejection, sadness and anger
- the burden of responsibility of taking on the carer role
- living with stigma and fear.

It must be emphasised, however, that problematic drug use does not necessarily mean that parents will lack parenting skills and be 'bad parents'. What usually happens is that the drug problem disrupts family functioning and it is this disruption which leads to longer term difficulties.

There are differences between the way individual family members deal with, or are affected by, drug use in the family, depending on their role and position in the family, their gender and their relationship to the user.

- Parents are initially more shocked than siblings, who may already be aware of the drug use.
- Siblings may conceal the drug use to minimise the effect it may have on the rest of the family. Siblings may very often be resentful of the attention the drug-using member of the family is attracting, resulting in conflict and animosity. The siblings of drug users may be at more risk of using drugs themselves.
- Fathers can be less likely to seek support and can display a much more aggressive and judgemental attitude towards the drug user.
- Partners may experience greater levels of verbal and physical abuse.

■ The needs of families

The effects of drug use on families create a range of needs. These needs are by no means universal and so will require a variety of responses, services and support. Adfam's report, *Families in Focus*,[4] produced as a result of consultation with family members, provides a rich picture of the perceptions and the needs of families affected by drugs and alcohol. The following points are drawn from that report.

■ The need to cope with stigma

Families report the negative effects of dealing with stigma and the fact that this often prevents them from accessing support. Stigma also increases the likelihood of concealment. Prejudice is a major barrier in accessing services. Families report exclusion from primary care services, together with a self-inflicted exclusion arising from the fear of being judged.

■ The need to access services

Information about treatments and services is a top priority for families. Where services do exist, families often do not know about them or how to access them. This is particularly apparent in rural communities and in the provision of specialist support for families from diverse ethnic groups.

■ The need to be involved in the treatment process

Families reported anger and confusion about their exclusion from participation in the treatment provided to their family member. Some families spoke of being told that their child was 'in treatment' but with no explanation about what that treatment entailed or what they might expect to encounter when the child returned home. Failing to involve families in aftercare significantly reduces the likelihood that recovery will be sustained. Interestingly, this lack of information was felt by families in both inpatient and community-based settings.

One parent spoke of her anger when told by her teenage son about his visit to a harm reduction worker who taught him to smoke heroin rather than inject it. Whilst this is a valid harm reduction technique, failing to explain to the significant others who surround the user what such an intervention is intended to achieve will reduce the likelihood of its being successful. Families felt that workers were hiding behind confidentiality when they could have provided general information about treatment for families. Anecdotal evidence suggests that some treatment providers expect staff to deal with both the user and their families, placing that staff member in a difficult (and sometimes impossible) situation.

Many families believe that treatment is the answer for the user, the magic bullet. This, of course, may well be so for many users but not for all and this reality can be difficult for families, particularly parents, to cope with. Waiting times for treatment are a source of frustration for families, believing that if only treatment could be accessed immediately all their problems would be solved. Families may also ascribe treatment relapse to a lack of support from agencies, resulting in a further barrier between the source of support and the family.

■ The need for a range of support services for families affected by drugs

Since families have a range of needs, so they will require a variety of responses, services and support. Once again, these vary from area to area and are by no means universal or standardised.

Some areas have few drugs services of any kind, let alone specialist services for families. Where such services exist, they do so because of the support of a local commissioner with a particular interest in this work, rather than through a planned strategy. Neither do many of the current services receive long-term funding; this means that large amounts of time and money are spent on seeking follow-on funding, rather than investing in quality of service provision.

Informal consultation with community groups and practitioners in the families field and the drugs field reveals a common agreement that there is a need to extend and enhance support for families and that this support should be standardised.

This need has been identified at a national, strategic level. The government's updated Drug Strategy[5] cites the following target: 'Parents, carers and families will have greater access to advice, help, counselling and mutual support in relation to drug misuse'. One of the strategy's objectives for preventing problematic drug use among young people is by 'improving services for parents and carers by setting clear standards for the support offered to parents who are concerned about substance misuse or whose family members have a problem'. The National Treatment Agency's *Models of Care* recognises that 'The needs of carers and families must also be considered in line with the Carer (Recognition & Services) Act, 1995'.[6]

Families require emotional, social and practical support. Emotional support can be accessed from informal sources such as friends and relatives or from more formal sources such as:

- self-help groups
- facilitator-led support groups
- telephone and online support
- one-to-one support
- befriending
- family therapy and counselling.

Practical support can meet the needs of families by providing:

- information on current treatments and information about drugs, via printed and website material
- alternative therapies, stress and relaxation techniques to cope with anxiety
- training on managing stress
- aftercare support (when formal treatment has finished)
- advocacy
- access to respite
- assistance with childcare
- financial advice
- health information.

Families also may have some very specific needs associated with drug use: for example, those families coping with a user with a dual diagnosis or with HIV or hepatitis C. Harm reduction advice is particularly important to minimise the risk of transmission of HIV and hepatitis C within the home.

■ The advantages of involving families

The advantages and benefits of providing support and services for families affected by drugs include social, emotional and health benefits and strategic and financial benefits.

The social, emotional and health benefits include:

- helping families to recognise their own needs and seek help
- improving communication within the family
- reducing isolation and anxiety
- identifying and addressing family issues.

There is evidence[1] that involving families in drug treatment, and particularly in the critical period of aftercare, improves treatment outcomes:

- by increasing support for the drug user
- by improving the family's understanding of drugs and drug treatment
- by creating a common goal for the treatment agency, drug user and family, for example, a realistic expectation of treatment outcomes.

Many of the families Adfam consulted were eager to participate actively in treatment but in England, no examples were found where direct family involvement in treatment or aftercare occurs.[4] It must be noted, however, that not all drug users wish to involve their families in treatment, because they no longer have any contact with their family, they believe their family would desire different treatment outcomes – for example, abstinence rather than maintenance – or they wish their drug use to remain a secret from their family.

There are strategic and financial benefits of families supporting drugs users.

- Family support costs for services are non-existent or very low – they are an unpaid workforce. However, unpaid is not necessarily without cost; families often suffer loss of earnings, debt and loss of employment through caring for a drug user.
- Families are in abundant supply.
- There is a high availability and flexibility of family support – 24 hours a day, seven days a week.
- Families are not subject to some of the restrictions which apply to formal organisations and can concentrate on service delivery.
- Families can offer a long-term commitment.
- Families have specialist knowledge of the individual drug user.
- Families usually have a high degree of investment in the individual and are motivated towards a successful outcome.
- Families are an untapped resource of a range of skills and have easy access to the individual.

■ The role of primary healthcare

Unfortunately, Adfam's research revealed reports of families who had failed to find help at their general practitioners. Even though many went to their GP first in search of help, all too often they reported that the GP response was to offer the family member medication to cope with their stress. As one mother said, 'I've had enough Prozac; what I want is help'. In addition, we heard a few, distressing reports of entire families who had been excluded from their local surgeries because a family member was using drugs problematically. In one such case, a young mother with four children whose partner was using heroin was excluded from the surgery nearest her, forcing her to walk with her four children some miles across the city to find primary care.

A British study[7,8] has shown the feasibility and potential of a general practice intervention to improve coping and relieve stress among family members affected by a family member's drug use. Given a coherent programme and ongoing support, primary care staff can be recruited and trained to work with families of drug users whose coping and health can be improved by a relatively brief intervention which need not involve the doctor. Relatives thus strengthened should be in a better position to facilitate the user's treatment. It is interesting, although not surprising, to note that many more women than men participate in such initiatives, raising the issue of whether to tailor interventions for mothers and wives or to do more to recruit men. It may be realistic to accept the primary role of women and to use them as ways to access male family members.

Policy, practice and remuneration strategies need to acknowledge the critical role primary care plays in the support of families affected by problem drug use. To match this, attitudes towards supporting families need to change so primary care teams recognise both the vital role they play in the treatment of drug misuse and their need for emotional and practical support in their own right.

Key points

- Families of drug users require significant support in their own right, to deal with the myriad problems they experience.
- There is growing evidence that there are advantages in involving families in drug treatment, including an improvement in treatment outcomes.
- The first access point for family support is usually the GP.
- There is a need to increase the number of support services for families and these services should be as diverse as the needs of the families themselves.

■ References

1 Stanton M and Todd T (1982) *The Family Therapy of Drug Abuse and Addiction*. Guilford Press, New York.

2 Velleman R, Bennet G, Miller T *et al.* (1993) The families of problem drug users: a study of 50 close relatives. *Addiction*. **88**: 1281–9.

3 Svenson LW, Forster DI, Woodhead SE *et al.* (1995) Individuals with a chemical dependent family member. Does their healthcare increase? *Canad Fam Physician*. **41**: 1488–93.

4 Adfam (2002) *Families in Focus*. Adfam, London.

5 Home Office (2002) *Updated Drug Strategy*. Home Office, London.

6 National Treatment Agency (2002) *Models of Care for Treatment of Adult Drug Users*. NTA, London. Available online at: www.nta.nhs.uk

7 Capello A, Templeton L, Krishnan M *et al.* (2000) A treatment package to improve

primary care services for relatives of people with alcohol and drug problems. *Addiction Res.* **8**: 471–84.
8 Capello A, Orford J, Velleman R *et al.* (2000) Methods for reducing alcohol and drug related family harm in non-specialist settings. *J Mental Health (UK)*. **9**: 329–43.

■ Further reading

- Bancroft A, Carty A, Cunningham-Burley S *et al.* (2002) *Support for the Families of Drug Users: a review of the literature.* Scottish Executive Drug Misuse Research Programme, Edinburgh.
- Home Office (2003) *Hidden Harm. Responding to the needs of children of problem drug users.* Stationery Office, London.
- MacDonald D, Russell P, Bland N *et al.* (2002) *Supporting Families and Carers of Drug Users: a review.* Scottish Executive Drug Misuse Research Programme, Edinburgh.

■ Useful contacts

Adfam
The national organisation committed to making sure that families affected by drugs and alcohol receive the help they need. Adfam's website gives details of local support on www.adfam.org/uk
Helpline: 0207 928 8898

FRANK
National drugs helpline on 0800 77 66 00 and www.talktofrank.com

PADA (Parents Against Drug Abuse)
Information, support and services for parents of drug users.
Helpline: 08457 02 38 67
www.btinternet.com/~padahelp/

CHAPTER 13

Practical aspects of managing drug users

Judy Bury

Many healthcare staff anticipate that the behaviour of people with drug dependence using their service will be difficult. Many GPs are willing to work with drug users but may become disillusioned by a sense of failure or because of the problems that drug users sometimes cause for the practice. They may feel untrained and uncertain about how to deal with these patients, who can be very challenging. This chapter suggests some strategies for avoiding situations that may give rise to difficult behaviour.

■ Implications for the practice

Caring for drug users in general practice can cause problems for the primary care team and disruption to the running of the practice.

- Drug users can be difficult and demanding and working with them can be stressful. The rewards may be poorly understood and may not be immediately evident.
- Caring for drug users may cause disagreements between individual doctors and between doctors and other staff as ideological and procedural differences are exposed.
- Staff and other patients may be upset by the behaviour of some drug users.

A practice faced with the task of providing care for drug users will find the work easier and more fulfilling if it invests time exploring and acknowledging these issues. Many of these problems can be prevented by combining compassionate care with the setting of limits on behaviour.

■ Questions to consider as a practice team

1 Does the practice have an ethos relating to its care of drug users?
2 Do local fellow professionals have an understanding of the service your practice is able to offer to drug users?

3 What would be the experience of a patient seeking an appointment at your practice to discuss their drug dependence?
4 What protocols and standards for behaviour should your practice develop to minimise the risk of misunderstanding and conflict with drug-using patients?

■ Setting limits on behaviour: the use of practice policies and agreements

> Doctor A has been working with drug users for six years but does not feel he is getting anywhere. He fears he has been conned and worries that drugs prescribed by him are being sold on the street. His partners think he is too soft with drug users and object to seeing his patients when he goes on holiday. On returning from holiday, he finds that four drug-using patients he was treating have been taken off the practice list in his absence. This leads to discussions within the practice about establishing a practice policy for dealing with drug users. Doctor A is encouraged to apply firmer limits to the behaviour of his drug-using patients while the other doctors agree to become more involved and to discuss the management of difficult patients rather than automatically taking them off the list.

Some GPs are reluctant to apply firm limits to the behaviour of drug users, believing that to do so would damage the doctor–patient relationship. In fact, this is far from being the case. Drug users have often lacked parenting, or at least appropriate parenting, and may be stuck in adolescent behaviour. In order to mature, they need care and concern on the one hand and firm and consistent boundaries on the other. In order to provide such boundaries, practices may benefit from an agreed written policy about working with drug users. GPs should consider using individual agreements with drug users so that they are made aware of the policies of the practice and can be reminded of them when they forget. When drug users break the individual agreement, the appropriate sanction (e.g. warning, withdrawal of prescription, removal from list) should be applied consistently. Using such policies and agreements and applying sanctions in a consistent manner reduces the disruption caused by drug users to the running of a practice. It is also beneficial for the drug user as it encourages maturation.

■ Practice policies

It is helpful for GPs in a practice to agree on certain aspects of working with drug users or to agree to disagree. For example, in some practices all the GPs may be willing to see and/or prescribe for drug users whilst in others it may be agreed that only some of the GPs will do this work. It is always helpful for each drug user to see only a named GP (and a named deputy in his or her absence) to encourage continuity of care and to discourage 'shopping around' between different GPs in the practice. The practice may wish to decide on policies relating to appointments, prescriptions and medication and to define what they consider to be acceptable and unacceptable behaviour. These can then be written down and reviewed from time to time. There are many different kinds of practice policy; it is for each practice to decide what seems appropriate and then to be consistent in its application.

It is useful to involve practice staff in discussions about the formulation of a practice policy. At the very least, once the practice policy has been agreed between the doctors, it is important to discuss it with any practice staff who might be involved in its implementation, especially receptionists, so that they are familiar with it and can raise any concerns about its application.

Issues to consider when formulating a practice policy

Appointments

Do you wish to have a named doctor for each drug user?

Do you have a policy about:
- patients arriving without an appointment?
- patients arriving late for an appointment?
- patients asking for home visits to discuss medication?
- patients wishing to discuss their medication on the phone?

Prescriptions and medication

What is your policy on:
- replacing lost prescriptions?
- replacing lost medication?
- releasing medication early?
- prescription arrangements for going on holiday?

Behaviour

What is your attitude to drug users attending appointments accompanied by a group of friends?

What action should be taken in the event of:
- patients shouting at receptionists or other patients?
- patients threatening receptionists or other patients?
- patients being violent?

What are the situations in which the receptionist should:
- call a doctor?
- call the police?

Have the doctors agreed how they will respond to a call from a receptionist?

■ The importance of consistency

The receptionists in practice B have been encouraged to be firm with drug users. Each drug user has been told that they will not be seen without an appointment. A drug user is demanding to be seen and the receptionist has stated clearly that he has to make an appointment. The drug user continues to demand to be seen. A GP comes out of her room, approaches the reception desk and invites the drug user into her room. The drug user emerges five minutes later holding a prescription which he waves triumphantly at the receptionist, who feels undermined and put down.

Once a practice policy has been agreed, it is important to be consistent in its application. If receptionists are expected to be firm in their application of the policy, it is important that they are supported and backed up. If a receptionist is interpreting the policy inappropriately, this should be discussed with him or her after the event, preferably involving the practice manager. If the policy is found to be inappropriate (for example, it may emerge that there are occasions when drug users can be seen without an appointment) then the policy should be reviewed and, if necessary, changed.

In the above scenario, familiar in most practices working with drug users, if the receptionist was interpreting the policy correctly yet the GP felt that she had to intervene, perhaps to avoid distress to other patients, she could back up the receptionist by approaching the patient and reinforcing what the receptionist has said, e.g. 'Now, you know you can't be seen without an appointment, so let's see when the next appointment is available'. Alternatively, the GP can take the patient to her room to reinforce this message. (Some practices have a 'hassle' room – perhaps an interview room or an area off the waiting room – where upset, angry or disruptive patients can be dealt with away from the public view of the waiting area.) In either case, it is important for the GP to talk to the receptionist afterwards to support them in what they were doing and to explain what actions she has taken and why, e.g. 'You were handling that fine; I just came to bail you out because the noise was beginning to disturb other people. You'll be pleased to know that I reinforced what you were saying and sent him away without a prescription'.

■ Breaking and reviewing practice policies

Inevitably, even with the most clearcut policy, there will be occasions when a GP feels that the situation warrants contravening the policy. Unexpected events such as family bereavements may necessitate prescriptions being issued early or without an appointment. It would obviously be insensitive and inappropriate for the GP to apply the policy rigidly in all circumstances. The term 'flexible rigidity' describes the approach that works best.

If a doctor feels that there are reasons why it is necessary to break the practice policy and give the patient a prescription without an appointment, it is important that he or she goes back to the receptionist afterwards to explain the reason for this.

Some practices find it helpful to have a forum for the GPs to share with one another occasions on which they have found it necessary to go against the policy. This then allows the GPs to recognise if there are certain drug users who are regularly persuading them to bend the rules and/or if there are one or more GPs who find it difficult to apply the policy. It is also important to review the policy itself from time to time (perhaps annually) and involve all the staff in a discussion about how the policy is working and whether it needs to be changed. If a significant event has occurred involving the behaviour of a drug-using patient, the team can learn from this by using a critical event analysis format to reinforce or adapt the policy.

■ Learning to say 'no'

A drug user is consulting Doctor C about a long-standing drug problem. She has run out of her prescribed drugs before her next prescription is due. The GP has refused to issue the prescription early but the drug user continues to ask for her drugs. For a while the GP continues to state that he will not give her the prescription but, as she continues to ask, the GP's resolve weakens and he says 'Well, all right then, just this once' and writes out the prescription.

There is no doubt that some GPs find it difficult to say 'no' to patients. They may find this particularly difficult if they have built up a relationship with a troublesome patient over a period of time and have persuaded themselves that it is appropriate to prescribe out of compassion and concern for that patient. It is important for the GP to know that giving in to the patient is often not helpful. Just as with an adolescent, it can be quite undermining and unsettling for the patient if no limits are applied to his or her behaviour. Sometimes a GP starts by saying 'no' but, as in the scenario above, gives in after a while. Unfortunately, this may give the message to the patient that if they nag for long enough then they will get what they want. If a GP is able to say 'no' and stick to this, the drug user may verbally abuse the GP at the time but will ultimately benefit from this application of limits. The drug user may even return and thank the doctor for his or her firmness!

Just as firmness without care and concern is unlikely to be helpful to the drug user, so care and concern without firmness are unlikely to be helpful either. Firmness also has the added advantage that it is likely to contribute to the smooth running of the practice.

This approach may be appropriate for a range of patients apart from drug users, for example the patient who repeatedly requests inappropriate home visits or the patient who is reluctant to come off hypnotics. By employing this approach with drug users, GPs may increase their confidence in applying it with other patients. Involving staff members in taking a team approach to working with drug users can enhance the working of the practice team. Thus, learning to work effectively with drug users can bring benefits to the practice as a whole.

■ Agreements or contracts

Once a practice policy has been agreed, an agreement or contract for the individual drug user can be drawn up to explain the policy of the practice with regard to appointments and prescriptions and to set out for the drug user guidelines about appropriate and inappropriate behaviour. An agreement can be used to underline that the patient is entering a treatment programme which will have benefits to them and which will regularly review goals. It can be used to highlight particular areas of concern that may include the safe storage of Controlled Drugs after they have been dispensed or the need for regular urine toxicity testing. Written agreements allow the drug user to make sense of the boundary setting that is implicit in the agreement.

As with policies, there are different types of agreement, as their contents will depend on the particular circumstances of the practice and the policy that has been agreed. It is helpful, however, if the agreement indicates what sanctions will be applied if the agreement is broken and if these sanctions are not too specific. It is more helpful if the agreement says 'Your prescription *may* be stopped' or 'You *may* be removed from the practice list' rather than 'You *will* be ...', thus allowing for a degree of flexibility. It is, however, helpful to indicate if there are any 'absolute' offences, where flexibility will not be exercised. For example, a practice may decide that any violence to staff or to other patients or any theft of prescriptions or prescription pads will always result in removal from the list. If so, this should be indicated in the agreement.

Some practices have found it helpful to explain the situation to the drug user in terms of 'yellow card' and 'red card' offences, as in football. Thus, the breaking of some rules, such as repeatedly being late for appointments, might lead to a warning – a 'yellow card' – but if the drug user continues to break these rules in spite of the warning, then a 'red card' might apply; that is, the prescription may be stopped. Certain behaviour, such as violence or theft, may lead to an immediate 'red card'; that is, stopping the prescription or removal from the practice list.

■ Using agreements in the practice

> Two drug users are sitting in the waiting room of practice D. One is obviously intoxicated and from time to time shouts at the receptionist, asking how much longer she must wait. The other is accompanied by a group of friends some of whom are addressing other patients and using bad language.

It is simpler to have a standard agreement to which extra clauses can be added than to write out an agreement from scratch with each drug user. If a standard agreement is used, then the receptionists can be made aware of who is on an agreement. This can be very helpful to them in enforcing rules about certain aspects of behaviour. Thus the receptionist can say to a drug user 'You know that your medication can't be replaced' or, as in the above scenario, 'You know that you're not meant to come with lots of friends. I'm afraid they'll have to wait outside'.

The terms of the agreement can be discussed when the drug user is started on a prescription. This provides an opportunity for the drug user to ask questions, clarify any uncertainties and indicate whether they feel that the terms of the agreement are reasonable. The drug user is then asked to sign the agreement, which is also signed by the GP. A copy can be kept in the notes and a copy given to the drug user. It can be referred back to in the future and the drug user reminded of its contents, especially if problems arise. Using an agreement in this way can encourage adult behaviour.

An example of an agreement is given here. A version of this is employed in a number of practices and practices are encouraged to adapt it for their own use.

Example of an agreement

Name: ....   Date: ....

Doctors, staff and many patients have been upset by the behaviour of some surgery attenders. Many of these people are attending for prescriptions of addictive drugs. You are now receiving a regular prescription for addictive medication and we require you to accept these rules.

Behaviour
1 I agree to attend appointments promptly and quietly.
2 I agree not to upset the receptionists or other patients in the waiting room.
3 Due to restriction of space in the waiting room, I agree to attend my appointments unaccompanied whenever possible.

Behaviour outside these limits may result in the receptionists or doctors asking you to leave the surgery premises. If necessary, the police will be called and you may be removed from the practice list and no longer be seen at this surgery.

Prescription, medication and appointment
1 I agree to be responsible for making my appointments and checking that my appointment is correct in our appointment book.
2 I accept responsibility for turning up for my appointment on time.
3 I agree to attend only the doctors mentioned below, on this form, and to discuss my prescription only with them.
4 I agree not to use emergency appointments or house calls to discuss my prescription.
5 I agree to be responsible for my prescription and medication and recognise that these cannot be replaced.
6 I agree that no alteration will be made to my prescription without my own doctor's permission.

My doctor is Dr: His/her half-day is:

....

In his/her absence I will consult Dr...

I HAVE READ THE ABOVE RULES, I UNDERSTAND WHAT THEY MEAN, I AGREE TO ABIDE BY THEM AND REALISE THAT IF I DO NOT, MY PRESCRIPTION MAY BE STOPPED AND THAT I MAY BE REMOVED FROM THE DOCTOR'S MEDICAL LIST.

Signature: ....   Date:....................................
(Patient)

Signature: ....   Date:....................................
(Doctor)

■ Case conferences

Particularly difficult patients or situations benefit from being shared by more than one professional and a consultation can be arranged between the GP, drug user, their drug worker or any other person from the practice team, to agree a written way forward for that individual. Sharing difficult decisions in this way can help to defuse a contentious situation, reinforce boundaries of acceptable behaviour, redefine the goals of treatment, illustrate a consistency of approach and demonstrate to the patient that you care about the outcomes of their treatment.

■ Some practical hints

Apart from the use of policies and agreements, there are other practical points that can assist in the management of drug users in general practice.

■ Appointments

Many unemployed drug users are semi-nocturnal, staying awake until early morning and sleeping in late. Early appointments are unlikely to be kept.

Care by receptionists in ensuring that they and the patient have correctly noted the appointment time may save later confrontation. The use of cards as in hospital outpatient departments is found to be helpful by some practices.

Many practices now have the ability to make appointments by computer while the patient is in the consultation. It can be helpful for the GP to make the next appointment for the drug user to coincide with their next prescription and to give this to the patient before they leave.

■ Behaviour

The use of an 'incident book' for receptionists to record details of patients behaving in a disruptive manner may serve both as a warning and as a way of assessing problems encountered. It is important that the entries in the incident book are reviewed on a regular basis, that appropriate action is taken and documented and that feedback is given to the staff involved in the incident about the action taken and the reasons for this. Sometimes, however, simply opening the book and asking for the patient's name can be enough to defuse the situation – perhaps because the drug user is reminded of school!

Although, in theory, putting a glass panel between the receptionists and patients increases the receptionists' sense of security, many practices have found that the behaviour of patients improves if such panels are removed. Behaviour often also improves if the waiting area is enlarged or made brighter.

Practices might want to consider the installation of panic buttons in the reception area and/or in surgeries. Local funding is often available for this. If installed, it is essential that GPs and staff are all clear about what action to take in the event that the alarm is activated.

■ Drug user clinics

GPs may wish to consider seeing all or some of their drug-using patients at a special clinic session. The main advantage of this approach is that drug users are not mixing with and potentially upsetting other patients in the waiting room and that the doctor can work in collaboration with a drug counsellor. The main disadvantages stem from the potentially disruptive effects of bringing drug users together in a group. In most instances, drug users benefit more from the effects of normalising their behaviour by being seen during an ordinary surgery.

Many drug users are sensitive to the actual or perceived attitudes of doctors or healthcare staff towards them. Treated with courtesy and consideration, most respond in kind.

Key points

- Many strategies are available to reduce the risk of difficult behaviour.
- Implications of caring for drug users should be discussed by the whole practice team.
- Many problems can be prevented by combining compassionate care with setting limits.
- The use of practice policies and individual agreements can help with limit setting.

■ Acknowledgement

Any improvements in this chapter since the first edition are due to the wise additions suggested by my colleague David Ewart, who has extensive experience of caring for drug users in general practice in Edinburgh.

CHAPTER 14

The primary care team and shared care

Jim Barnard, Jean-Claude Barjolin and Christina McArthur

General practice has been playing an increasingly important role in the delivery of treatment for drug dependency, usually through 'shared-care' schemes. This has been formalised in the national framework for the commissioning of treatment for drug users, *Models of Care*, published in October 2002 jointly between the Department of Health and the National Treatment Agency.[1] *Models of Care* describes a four-tier treatment system in which services are characterised by different thresholds of access, specialism and complexity of intervention (*see* Chapter 15). General practitioners providing treatment for drug dependency are part of tier 3 services, loosely described as 'community-based prescribing'. All GPs should also be providing tier 1 general medical services (GMS) and many will provide tier 2 (e.g. harm reduction support, advice and information).

There is a growing evidence base for the effectiveness and safety of treating drug users in general practice.[2,3] There is now a specific government target for 30% of GPs to be involved in shared care[4] as part of the government's broader initiative to reduce waiting times and expand treatment.[5] At the time of writing, 23% of GPs are involved.[6]

The term 'shared care' was defined by the Department of Health in 1995 as 'the joint participation of general practitioners and specialists in the delivery of care for people with a drug misuse problem'.[7] This no longer adequately describes the range of services and different models for delivering treatment that have developed in primary care. 'Primary care-based treatment' is now a more useful term to use because, as described below, services are no longer purely delivered within traditional shared-care models. There is considerable variation between localities and even between practices in the way services are provided.[8] However, models tend to fall into one of two broad types – traditional shared care or intermediate services. There is likely to be more homogeneity in the future with the implementation of National Enhanced Services (NES) under the new GP Contract[9] and the clearer definition of competencies which will be associated with the roles of the generalist/NES GP, the GP with a special clinical interest (GPwSI) and the GP working in the role of specialist.

Key principles for developing primary care-based treatment

- Appropriate support (e.g. drug worker, GPwSI), depending on local need and GP experience.
- Appropriate remuneration in line with the new GP Contract or separately contracted-for intermediate services.
- Ownership by primary care, through involvement in planning and development.
- Clear care/referral pathways.
- Safety – robust local guidelines and protocols, supervision within a local clinical governance framework.
- Competency – training for all GPs and primary care-based staff to an appropriate level.
- Adequate arrangements for continuing professional development (CPD) and appraisal (*see* Chapter 17).

■ How primary care-based treatment is delivered

■ Traditional shared-care models

GP support comes from NHS trust or non-statutory services, either of a specialist nature or increasingly a community-based prescribing service headed by a GPwSI. Schemes vary widely around the country, from formalised and structured to informal arrangements. In future they will probably be delivered as a National Enhanced Service (NES) under the new GP Contract. The level of GP involvement within these schemes is dependent on both the scheme itself and the experience and expertise of the GP. Historically some GPs have treated drug users without support. This is not recommended and is becoming more unusual as agreed clinical governance procedures are becoming the norm.

GP liaison service

GP support comes from NHS trust, PCT or non-statutory services, in the form of a GP liaison worker. Usually the responsibility for the initial assessment and initiation into treatment resides with the clinical specialist and the GP liaison worker. Once stable, the client is referred back to the GP. The patient, the GP and drug liaison worker work together to formulate a care plan that is reviewed regularly.

With good support from the GP liaison worker, larger numbers of drug users can be seen in general practice and drug users have good access to general medical services. However, in some places the role of the GP has been reduced to little more than signing the prescription, which may hamper the development of additional skills for the GP and militates against primary care ownership of the service.

Primary care facilitation service

A dedicated team or project, with a remit to develop and sustain shared care alongside existing local services. A GPwSI (or another experienced professional) is appointed to act as GP facilitator. There may be additional dedicated staff to manage the project and co-ordinate training and development. A named shared-care co-ordinator visits and supports local GPs and establishes referral and shared-care arrangements with local services. GPs may sign up to a local contractual arrangement which includes:

- prescribing protocols
- a shared-care protocol specifying referral arrangements, role of different agencies, support available such as client assessment, urine testing and rapid referral back into specialist service when necessary
- locally dedicated GP support workers
- clinical audit
- regular training and CPD
- annual GP facilitator review visit to GP
- payment for GPs working to agreed protocols within the scheme.

This may be a more expensive way to deliver services but it allows for the implementation of robust clinical governance frameworks and primary care has access to high levels of support both clinically and strategically.

■ Intermediate services

Service from GPs with a special interest (GPwSI)

GPs within this model will have greater levels of interest, training and expertise in the substance misuse field than a generalist GP. They have usually completed the RCGP certificate course or equivalent, as well as a commitment to at least 15 hours continuing professional development (CPD) in substance misuse every year.[10] They will normally be able to manage more complex problems, offer support and supervision to generalists and may be contracted to offer services to patients not on their practice list. They may lead a community-based prescribing service providing an intermediate level between generalist GP services and the specialist service. This service would treat people whose GP does not provide a service for drug dependency and/or those with problems that are deemed too complex for generalist GPs. GPwSIs may also be commissioned to play a supportive and developmental role with generalist GP services (*see* above) and will usually be involved with the shared-care monitoring group. It is recommended that GPwSIs receive supervision from a specialist in substance misuse.[10]

Case example

Two GPs were commissioned to run a service aimed at rapidly increasing access to treatment for local drug users. They took on drug users from specialist services who were deemed stable but whose own GP wouldn't prescribe and drug users newly referred for treatment. They were able to manage most of these, rather than referring on to specialists. They encouraged patients' own GPs to take over treatment for their patients once stabilised. They developed local guidelines and protocols and more than doubled the amount of substitute prescribing in the locality. Patients were mostly managed by the GP and only referred to a drug worker if there was a specific need (about 25% of cases). The service has reduced waiting times and achieved impressive outcomes.

Practices serving specialist populations

These are usually salaried GPs working within a PMS with a remit to treat particular populations including drug users or homeless people. They can generally be found in areas where there are gaps in local service delivery. PMS practices (and other intermediate services) can provide a pragmatic, short-term solution to treatment capacity problems. PMS practices often provide low-threshold access to general healthcare and drug dependency treatment. They can treat a large number of people and sometimes employ their own drug support worker.

It is important to gain the support of local GPs to facilitate the reintegration of drug users into mainstream general practice so that patients do not remain forever in a 'drug' practice.

Case example

Two PMS practices working together with a remit for substance misuse have more than 100 people actively in treatment (a larger number than the specialist service locally). The practices employ a specialist drug worker who is also attached to a non-statutory agency, as well as a specialist health visitor. One GP in the practice has a special clinical interest and provides clinical support for colleagues. The PMS has created the capacity to meet local demand. The practices also cater for a large general practice population, thus overcoming the problems of being a 'drug practice'. However, the GPs have difficulty referring into the specialist service if a patient proves too complex due to the specialist service policy of not taking on patients who were not initially treated by them prior to treatment in primary care.

■ How to avoid pitfalls

Pitfalls can be avoided if the key principles described earlier are adhered to. Whatever the scheme or type of GP involvement, appropriate levels of support for services, training, supervision and appropriate remuneration for the work contracted are necessary. A robust clinical governance framework should be in place, including joint protocols and clear referral pathways, to ensure medico-legal safety. Perhaps most importantly, primary care ownership for the scheme needs to be developed, ideally with peer leadership. Ownership can be achieved through meaningful engagement of primary care in the shared-care monitoring group (*see* below).

Case example

An area had developed all its prescribing services to be provided by GPs. This was largely due to the efforts and support of the local, well-respected drug service manager. However, there were no structured training for GPs, no local protocols, no GP involvement in planning and development, no reimbursement and no local agreement with the LMC. The local drug-using population increased and became more unstable as a sizeable travelling community moved into the area. GPs became uncomfortable prescribing large amounts of methadone and felt unsafe on medicolegal grounds. As a result, the LMC felt the situation was unacceptable and advised all GPs locally to give three months' notice to stop prescribing. This duly happened and a specialist clinic had to be set up within three months, which immediately had a waiting list of over a year. Significant levels of primary care involvement have still not been redeveloped in this locality.

The responsibility for ensuring that a comprehensive primary care-oriented treatment service is available in each locality rests with the drug action team and the shared-care monitoring group.[11]

The shared-care monitoring group

- A local strategic group set up to develop and monitor primary care-based treatment, as recommended in Department of Health Clinical Guidelines (1999).
- Organised by primary care trust or drug action team.
- Has high level of primary care membership including GPs, LMC, pharmacist and LPC representation. Has a primary care or PCT representative as chair.
- Should ensure all the necessary components for effective primary care treatment of drug users are set in place.
- For more information, *see* www.smmgp.co.uk

■ Support for GPs

■ Specialist clinical support

Generalist GPs will usually get their clinical support from a GPwSI or an addiction specialist. GPwSIs are recommended to get their supervision from a specialist. The definition of a specialist is problematic as there are very few qualified addiction psychiatrists nationally and in some areas the local 'specialist' may be a general psychiatrist who has agreed to take on the drug misuse brief and may be less knowledgeable and experienced than the GPwSI. Increasingly there are examples of GPs taking on the specialist role but although usually extremely experienced and able, they are not at present allowed to be formally recognised as addiction specialists.

Example checklist for dividing responsibilities within shared care

	Drug team		GP
Initial drug history assessment	(✓)		( )
Initial urine screen	( )	either	( )
Check for IV sites	( )	either	( )
Annual weighing	( )	either	( )
Prescribing	( )		(✓)
Titration of methadone dose	( )	either	( )
Pharmacy liaison	( )		(✓)
Database notification	( )	either	( )
Counselling	(✓)	both	(✓)
Random urine testing – at least six-monthly	( )	either	( )
HBV, HCV and HIV testing and counselling	( )	either	( )
Hepatitis A/B immunisation	( )	either	( )
Referral to secondary medical care	( )		(✓)
Sick certificate	( )		(✓)
Housing letters	(✓)		( )
Legal reports	( )	either	( )
Probation liaison	(✓)		( )
Rehabilitation referral	(✓)		( )
Detoxification referral	(✓)		( )
Social Services funding referral	(✓)		( )
Assistance with benefit problems	(✓)		( )
Child protection issues	(✓)	both	(✓)

NB: Division of responsibilities may vary locally and there may be others involved in such a checklist, for example pharmacists.

■ Drug worker support

In many instances the main support to general practice will be from a drug worker. Drug workers come from a variety of backgrounds such as nursing, social work or previous personal experience of drug use and treatment. They are usually referred to as GP liaison workers or primary care support workers. They are often employed by NHS trust substance misuse services although they may be employed by voluntary sector organisations or even directly by the PCT. Some practices, such as PMS practices, will employ drug workers directly.

The drug worker and the GP need to agree a division of responsibilities within the treatment process between them. This will usually be done with reference to local protocols, the experience of the GP and the amount of time the GP can devote to this area of work. Opposite is a checklist giving an example of division of responsibilities.

■ Other primary care-based staff

Practice nurses may choose to take a special interest in drug dependency treatment. Within the Department of Health there is a drive to create nurses with a special interest[12] and practice nurses are now able to access substance misuse training organised by the RCGP. Their role can vary from offering general healthcare and harm reduction, e.g. immunisation, sexual health advice, to supporting the treatment process itself.

Reception staff also have an important role to play as they are in the front line. If receptionists are welcoming and accepting of drug users, particularly those presenting for treatment for the first time, this will increase the likelihood of successful engagement in treatment. Training for reception staff can help to reduce conflict and enable the staff to understand and take pride in their role as well as contributing towards a good-quality treatment environment.[13] Reception staff need to feel supported by GPs and this is helped if all staff adhere to a practice agreement about how to manage drug users (*see* Chapter 13). When this happens, it is usual for reception staff to experience a good relationship with drug-using patients.

Practice administrative staff can also play an important role in co-ordinating information on drug users attending the surgery, especially if several GPs in a practice are providing treatment. For example, they can create a register of patients in treatment, draw the attention of the GP to patients who have not turned up for appointments, act as a link with the specialist services, co-ordinate prescriptions with the local pharmacies, cross-check that payments have been claimed for and received and supply data as required for the National Drug Treatment Monitoring Service and the PCT.

Pharmacists are pivotal to the successful delivery of primary care-based treatment and many are now developing a special interest in this field of work. The Centre for Pharmacy Postgraduate Education in association with the University of Manchester has developed an open learning pack for pharmacists in England[14] and some pharmacists have participated in the RCGP certificate course. The pharmacist has more regular contact with the patient than any other professional and can be particularly helpful in reporting back to the prescribing

GP any concerns about the well-being of the patient or possible inappropriate use of the prescription. Good relationships between GPs and pharmacists, understanding of roles and regular liaison are important.

In addition to dispensing, some pharmacists have taken on additional responsibilities such as providing needle exchange, harm reduction advice and supervised self-administration of methadone or buprenorphine. Increasingly pharmacists are being formally recognised as part of the treatment team. A well-known example is a 'four-way agreement' between the GP, the pharmacist, the patient and the drug worker in Berkshire.[15] Pharmacists are often active on the shared-care monitoring group and work with drug users is now being accepted as mainstream by some of the major pharmacy chains. One chain has even appointed regional representatives to promote the role of pharmacy in drug dependency treatment. Good communication between pharmacy and general practice is crucial in delivering the most effective treatment.

A robust clinical governance framework, including support from a shared-care co-ordinator, standard protocols and adequate training, is needed to ensure that the quality of service is of the same high standard no matter which pharmacy is providing it. It is important to remember that these additional services are not part of a pharmacist's core duties and that additional remuneration arrangements will be needed. It is likely that in future, services to drug users will be included as part of the new pharmacy contract which, at the time of writing, is being negotiated.

Pharmacist involvement in the planning of services is especially important as more innovative services are being set up. New services need not only to ensure that pharmacists are able to take on the increased workload but also to ensure that legal issues around the Misuse of Drugs Act are complied with.

As with GP reception staff, pharmacy staff play a crucial role in welcoming drug users and normalising their regular visits to the pharmacy whether for needle exchange or daily supervised consumption of substitute drugs.

Health visitors, midwives and district nurses may develop a special interest in drug use, particularly in PMS practices. Community nurses can be crucial in the identification of a drug or potential drug problem within a family and when handled sensitively can facilitate access into treatment. As providers of support to families and carers of drug users in and out of treatment, they are ideally placed to offer health education and harm reduction advice, all of which contributes to the effective management of drug users within the community.

■ RCGP training initiatives

In order to meet the training needs of GPs and other primary care professionals, the RCGP has developed a substance misuse training programme co-ordinated by a project team at the London Faculty. This is now divided into two parts.

■ RCGP Certificate Part 2

This is now well established and successful completion of the Certificate Part 2 is one of the ways in which GPs can demonstrate their competency to be a

GPwSI. It utilises a variety of educational methods and is now multidisciplinary. The programme requires a commitment to eight days of learning, including master classes, small group work and practical assignments.

■ RCGP Certificate Part 1

This is being developed as a course for generalists, to help GPs just beginning this work or to give some basic knowledge to GPs who want to learn a little about the topic. It will also enable GPs to meet the competencies for a generalist delivering a Locally Enhanced Service or, with more experience, a Nationally Enhanced Service (NES). It will prepare GPs for Part 2 of the Certificate, for those wanting to go on with developing their skills. It will be delivered in a blended learning package consisting of online and face-to-face training components. Other training resources and distance learning packages will be developed to support the Part 1 or provide learning options. Candidates who complete the course will receive a certificate of attendance.

■ Substance Misuse Management in General Practice network (SMMGP)

This is a national network for GPs and other primary care-based professionals interested in the treatment of drug dependency. It supports the development of high-quality treatment services, expertise and competence in a primary care setting. From small beginnings it has become a national resource for primary care. It produces a quarterly newsletter called *Network* and has a website with a range of useful resources, including examples of local guidelines, newsletter back issues and a very well-used interactive discussion forum where all issues pertaining to primary care-based treatment can be discussed.

Key points

- Primary care-based treatment has become increasingly diverse and the term 'shared care' no longer describes it adequately.
- The engagement of all those working in primary care, including pharmacists and reception staff, is necessary.
- Support, remuneration, clinical governance, training and primary care ownership are crucial.
- Shared-care monitoring groups should have active primary care input and ensure that local schemes meet the needs of primary care.
- There is now a *de facto* national service framework, nationally accredited training, a national GP Contract and a national primary care network.

■ References

1 National Treatment Agency (2002) *Models of Care for Treatment of Adult Drug Users.* NTA, London. Available online at: www.nta.nhs.uk

2 Gossop M, Marsden J, Stuart D *et al.* (1999) Methadone treatment practices and outcomes for opiate addicts treated in drug clinics and in general practice: results from the capital's national treatment outcome research study. *Br J Gen Pract.* **49**: 31–4.

3 Oliver P, Keen J, Rowse G *et al.* (2001) Deaths from drugs of abuse in Sheffield, 1998: the role of prescribed medication. *Br J Gen Pract.* **51**: 394–6.

4 Department of Health (2001) *The NHS Plan: deliverables for local modernisation reviews.* Stationery Office, London.

5 Stationery Office (1998) *Tackling Drugs to Build a Better Britain. The government's 10 year strategy for tackling drug misuse.* Stationery Office, London.

6 National Treatment Agency (2003) *Analysis of Drug Action Team Treatment Plan Returns.* NTA, London. Available online at: www.nta.nhs.uk

7 Department of Health (1995) *Reviewing Shared Care Arrangements for Drug Misusers.* EL (95) 114. Annex A. Department of Health, London.

8 Barnard J and Higson C (1999) Caring and sharing: modelling successful shared care. *Druglink.* **14**(1): 13–15.

9 British Medical Association, NHS Confederation (2003) *Investing in General Practice: the new General Medical Services Contract.* BMA/NHS Confederation, London. Available online at: www.bma.org

10 Department of Health, Royal College of General Practitioners (2003) *Guidelines for the Appointment of General Practitioners with Special Interests in the Delivery of Clinical Services – drug misuse.* Department of Health, London.

11 Department of Health (2000) *CLA Notification – additional funding for drug misuse services – annex E.* Department of Health, London.

12 Department of Health (2003) *Practitioners with Special Interests in Primary Care – implementing a scheme for nurses with special interests in primary care; liberating the talents.* Department of Health, London.

13 Carnwath T, Gabbay M and Barnard J (2000) A share of the action: GP involvement in drug misuse treatment in Greater Manchester. *Drugs Educ Prevent Policy.* **7**: 235–50.

14 Centre for Pharmacy Postgraduate Education (2002) *Opiate Treatment: supporting pharmacists for improved patient care – an open learning course for pharmacists.* Stationery Office, London.

15 Berkshire Substance Misuse Protocol Group (2001) *Management and Treatment of Substance Misuse in Berkshire.* Berkshire Healthcare NHS Trust, Reading.

■ Useful contact

Substance Misuse Management in General Practice (SMMGP)
www.smmgp.co.uk
Telephone: 0161 905 8581

orking with other agencies

Kate Davies and Jim Barnard

As previous chapters have described, many drug users can be and are managed within general practice, particularly with help and support from drug workers and counsellors. Sometimes it is necessary to refer drug users to other services for some or all of their care, although the GP will retain responsibility for meeting general healthcare needs.

Specialist service provision has until recently been patchy and inconsistent, with considerable variation from one district to another. The National Treatment Agency (NTA) was set up in April 2001 as a special health authority working with both the Department of Health and the Home Office to increase the availability, capacity and effectiveness of treatment for drug users in England. It aims to double the number of people in effective treatment, from 100 000 in 1998 to 200 000 in 2008, and to increase the proportion of people retained in or completing treatment year on year. These are key targets in the UK's 10-year strategy *Tackling Drugs to Build a Better Britain*.[1] The NTA has already had success in many areas in improving the distribution and quality of all types of drug service provision.

■ Drug and Alcohol Action Teams

Every area has a drug and alcohol action team (DAAT) or a drug action team (DAT), which commissions substance misuse services across their locality. There are 149 DATs in England working to treatment plans monitored by the NTA. They are partnership organisations which work closely with or are amalgamated with local crime and disorder reduction partnerships.

Funding for drug misuse treatment services for adults and, separately, for young people is allocated to DATs from the central government ring-fenced pooled budget for substance misuse prevention and treatment. Primary care trusts then act as bankers for the adult treatment budget and local authorities as bankers for the young people treatment budget. Additional funding comes from local partner organisations that are represented on the DAT, for example health, local authority, probation and police. Ideally this funding is also managed through the DAT and joint commissioning structures to allow the most effective deployment of the total sum available. The central government ring-fenced budget has been increasing significantly in recent years but contributions from local partner organisations may vary considerably from year to year.

Arrangements for funding and commissioning are organised differently in other parts of the UK outside England.

■ *Models of Care*

Models of Care[2] is a national framework for the implementation of quality standards for substance misuse services and is really a National Service Framework by another name. It sets out what is necessary to achieve equity, partnership, parity and consistency in the commissioning and provision of substance misuse treatment. Treatment provision is considered as a tier of services becoming more specialised as a user moves up the tiers.

- *Tier 1*: services not specifically for substance misusers but which come into contact with users. These should be able to offer information about services, low-level assessment and referral to treatment and harm reduction interventions. GMS for drug users would fit into this tier.
- *Tier 2*: open access drug and alcohol treatment services.
- *Tier 3*: structured community-based drug treatment services. These require the user to have a drug assessment and a care plan. Most community prescribing services are in this tier, together with psychological therapies, community detox and day-care programmes.
- *Tier 4*: residential services.

■ **Health and social care agencies**
■ **Street agencies**

The first point of referral for the GP will often be the local street agency or community drug team (CDT). Street agencies are almost all drop-in services provided by voluntary or non-statutory agencies based in the community. Often there is considerable overlap between street agencies and CDTs, which between them provide a wide range of services, usually in tier 2.

Services provided by street agencies

- Drop in, information, advice.
- Counselling – individual or group.
- Needle exchange.
- Safe sex advice and condom distribution.
- Complementary therapies.
- Outreach work.
- Referral to residential detox and rehabilitation facilities.
- Prescribing services (sometimes).
- Aftercare.

■ Community drug teams

Community drug teams are health service agencies set up in the late 1980s in response to the HIV epidemic, to work collaboratively with GPs by providing counselling and other services to drug users and supporting GPs in their prescribing role. CDTs or their equivalent now cover every locality in England. However, services have developed in such a way that CDTs are now often almost indistinguishable from drug dependency units (DDUs), which have adopted many of their characteristics. It is probably easier to abandon the distinction and just talk about services in terms of the *Models of Care* tiers which they deliver.

■ Drug dependency units

Drug dependency units (DDUs) were first established in the late 1960s and early 1970s. Because of the large increase in drug use in the 1980s, particularly in large cities, and the small number of DDUs, these services have been under tremendous pressure with long waits for users to be seen and accepted into treatment. This has been identified as one of the reasons why many referrals and first contacts do not lead to engagement in treatment.[3] In recent years, some new specialist units have been established, led by GPs, and in other units GPs have been appointed to positions previously held by consultant psychiatrists. Their philosophy is based on a key worker-led strategy for patients, with all but the most chaotic users maintained in general practice.[4] Nevertheless, in many areas a tension still exists between the rigid approach of the DDU (or CDT) to scripting and associated expectations of client behaviour, and the treatment style of local general practitioners who may quite appropriately impose fewer conditions on users for whom they are prescribing on a long-term basis. Clinic regimes and the conditions attached to treatment were common reasons given by a sample of opiate users who had never sought help from a DDU.[5]

This tension has contributed to the current situation in many areas of a mismatch between clients' needs and the services they are using. Complex and challenging users who 'fail' to keep to DDU/CDT rules end up being looked after in general practice whilst some stable users on a long-term script are taking up places on DDU/CDT programmes. These problems should be addressed by the implementation of *Models of Care*, particularly with the introduction of care co-ordination and integrated care pathways.

■ Crisis

Crisis may be associated with one or more of the following: acute intoxication, overdose, acute withdrawal or physical, psychiatric or social co-morbidities. Specialist crisis intervention services are rare and the GP will need to liaise with A and E departments, general medical and surgical services and the psychiatric service. GP 'out of hours' services may also be contacted by drug users and GP co-operatives and commercial deputising services should have a policy about how to respond appropriately to the kinds of problems which present at these times.

■ Psychiatric co-morbidity

'Dual diagnosis' is the term used to describe the status of drug users who have a concomitant mental health problem. There may be a causal, consequent or coincidental relationship between psychiatric morbidity and drug use. These patients are challenging to manage in psychiatric units, often because of behavioural problems. It may be difficult to get them admitted and for their drug use to be appropriately addressed when in hospital. They have low rates of compliance with aftercare. There is considerable interest in the psychiatric and drug addiction field in drawing up protocols for management of these patients. Correct diagnosis can often only be achieved after inpatient observation in a psychiatric unit. A local psychiatrist with an interest in drug addiction is an essential requirement but may not be available in all areas.

Patients with schizophrenic illness, manic depressive illness or severe depression often have their illness exacerbated by drug misuse. Patients defined as having personality disorder are often not helped by inpatient psychiatric therapy. Drug misuse may be a major factor in their care management. A decision must be made whether a community psychiatric nurse or a drug worker is the relevant key worker with overall responsibility for care management in patients with dual diagnosis.

■ Specialist inpatient detoxification

Inpatient drug misuse treatment services are available in a number of cities and towns. They provide medically supervised detoxification with counselling and support. Length of stay is usually four weeks. They may be particularly relevant for polydrug users with high levels of medical and psychiatric morbidity, although further research still needs to be done on effectiveness compared with detoxification in other settings.[6]

■ Secondary care services for physical co-morbidity

See Chapter 3.

■ Specialist obstetric care

See Chapter 10.

■ Residential rehabilitation

These services have been traditionally provided by voluntary agencies or non-statutory agencies. There are 70 centres in the UK offering 1279 places.[7] Over half provide or have access to detoxification facilities as well and most offer programmes of between three and nine months' duration. Funding for a place is organised through the community care budget of the Social Services department of the user's local authority of residence. A local community drugs worker can usually organise the referral and arrange for the necessary assessment and approval for funding. The availability of funding varies from place to place and from year to year and there may be long waits for admission. However, NTA waiting time requirements apply to residential rehabilitation and reductions in waiting times should be expected in the future.

Residential treatment programmes vary widely in concept and practice but fall broadly into four categories.[8]

1 The *concept house/therapeutic community* (Phoenix House is a well-known example). There is a strong reliance on the collective strength of peers and the value of intensive group work.
2 The *Christian rehabilitation house*, which may be strictly Christian (the resident must support the faith) or more loosely based on the Christian ethos which may motivate the staff but is not required of residents.
3 *Community integrated houses*, in which close links are formed with the local community and are seen as major elements within the rehabilitative process.
4 *Twelve-Step 'Minnesota model' houses*, based on the 12-Step programme of Narcotics Anonymous, which subscribes to the disease model of addiction and relies heavily on self-help techniques. NA subsequently provides continued support beyond the residential phase.

Despite these differences, residential centres share common features. Residents must be drug free and the centre provides a structured programme of psychological, educational and social therapy aimed at preparing the drug user to manage a drug-free life better when back in society. Users will generally have a feel for which type of rehab will suit their needs. More provision is needed for women, young people and people from black and minority ethnic groups.

Rehabilitation programmes may also be provided on a day-care basis.

■ Complementary therapies

Therapies such as hypnotherapy, shiatsu and acupuncture may be offered by drugs agencies as an adjunct or alternative to more conventional treatments. There is a scarcity of research data to support claims of effectiveness but these therapies are popular with users and they do apparently attract some drug users, e.g. cocaine users, into treatment services.[9]

■ Self-help networks

In its broadest sense, self-help refers to the support which drug users and their families and friends can draw on outside formal drug treatment. There is increasing encouragement from the NTA and DATs for users and carers to be involved in the commissioning, planning and delivery of services. As a result, there is a growing network of self-help family and carer support services, current and ex-user advocacy and support services. It is important for GPs to know about self-help networks for families, carers, users and ex-users, particularly any in existence locally.

■ Criminal justice treatment services

GPs may be asked to work in partnership with a number of different health and treatment services for substance misuse accessed through the criminal justice system.

■ Police

All police forces operate some form of arrest and referral scheme in conjunction with a local treatment provider. The aim is to exploit the opportunity of arrest to encourage drug users to enter treatment. The schemes vary from just offering contact numbers for drug treatment services to providing a more structured response, utilising drug workers on site or on call. Mandatory drug testing within custody suite settings is identifying high levels of heroin and crack/cocaine use in detainees.

Police surgeons, many of whom are also GPs, are involved in the assessment and treatment of drug users in police custody. They should take the opportunity to put drug users in contact with the appropriate treatment services, which may be best provided or co-ordinated by the GP.

■ Probation service

The probation service is now seen as a major partner, not only in the commissioning of specialist substance misuse services but also as a provider. The service is involved with Drug and Testing Treatment Orders (DTTOs), Absence Orders, prolific offender projects and a range of other criminal justice interventions such as arrest and referral, aftercare and resettlement packages.

When treating a drug user in general practice, it is useful to ask if he or she has a probation officer or is subject to a specific community sentence in relation to their substance misuse. Probation officers will see clients on a regular basis. It is helpful to them to know what treatment strategy a GP is following and they can provide useful feedback to the GP with their perception of how the user is coping. It is important to note that if the client is subject to a DTTO, they may already be on a prescribing programme.

■ Prison service

It is now considered important that drug users should receive a 'seamless service' while on remand or serving a sentence in prison. Counselling, Assessment, Referral Advice and Throughcare (CARATs) is now implemented in all prisons to ensure substance misuse service provision support and advice for prisoners. At the time of writing, much of prison healthcare is in the process of transferring from Home Office responsibility to that of the NHS. Prison health services have lagged behind those outside prison in terms of treatment provision for drug users and detoxification is very much more likely to be offered than maintenance treatment.

Discharge from prison can be a vulnerable time as tolerance may be reduced and the user may restart problematic drug use. General practitioners can help by offering emergency appointments for those discharged from prison on naltrexone medication so as to continue the medication without a break and not restarting pre-prison maintenance opiate medication without reassessment as reduced tolerance puts the user at risk of opiate overdose. There is still a need to improve the care pathways for aftercare and community integration once people leave prison and this is now a priority for all DATs under the criminal justice funding requirements.

■ Other services

GPs may also need to liaise with a number of other services including:

- housing departments
- supportive accommodation/supporting people housing networks
- welfare benefits advice
- education services
- employment services including services specifically set up to work with enabling substance misusers into employment (Progress2Work)
- young people's projects
- services for women such as help in dealing with domestic violence
- black and minority community projects
- Social Services departments, particularly children's services
- youth offending teams (in relation to under-19s).

When working within shared care, it is usually reasonable to expect the drug worker to organise these contacts. The local DAT should also be able to provide contact information for these services.

Key points

- Some drug users need to be managed by specialist drug treatment services, which are gradually improving in capacity and quality, although provision is still patchy.
- Many other agencies can provide useful support and help for the problems which drug users face and GPs need to be aware of how users can access these other agencies.
- The criminal justice system is increasingly becoming a route to treatment for drug users.
- Local drug action teams should have the power to improve local services and ensure gaps in services are filled.

■ References

1 Department of Health (1998) *Tackling Drugs to Build a Better Britain: the government's 10-year strategy for tackling drug misuse.* Stationery Office, London.
2 National Treatment Agency (2002) *Models of Care for Treatment of Adult Drug Users.* NTA, London. Available online at: www.nta.nhs.uk
3 National Treatment Agency (2002) *Making the System Work: waiting times guidance.* NTA, London.
4 Speed S and Janikievicz S (2000) Providing care to drug users on Wirral: a case study analysis of a primary health care/general practice-led drug service. *Drugs Educ Prevent Policy.* **7**(3): 257–77.
5 Bennett T and Wright R (1986) Opioid users' attitudes towards and use of NHS clinics, general practitioners and private doctors. *Br J Addiction.* **81**: 757–63.
6 Gossop M, Marsden J and Stewart D (2001) *National Treatment Outcome Research Study (NTORS) After 5 Years: changes in substance use, health and criminal behaviour during 5 years after intake.* National Addiction Centre, London.
7 Cooke C (1995) *Residential Rehabilitation. A report prepared for the Task Force to Review Services for Drug Misusers.* Department of Health, London.
8 Preston A and Malinowski A (1999) *The Rehab Handbook. A user's guide to rehab services and community care funding.* Drugscope, London.
9 National Treatment Agency (2002) *Treating Cocaine/Crack Dependence.* Research into Practice: 1a Drug Services' Briefing: Drug and alcohol findings. NTA, London.

■ Useful contacts

National Treatment Agency
Room 509
Hannibal House
Elephant & Castle
London SE1 6TE
Telephone: 0207 972 2226
www.nta.nhs.uk

Drugscope
32–6 Loman Street
London SE1 OEE
Information on drugs, library, news, services directory.
Telephone: 0207 928 1211
www.drugscope.org.uk

Narcotics Anonymous (NA)
UK Service Office
PO Box 1980
202 City Road
London EC1V 2PH
Self-help fellowship. Groups throughout UK.
Telephone: 0207 251 4007
Helpline: 0207 730 0009
www.ukna.org

Adfam National
Waterbridge House
32–6 Loman Street
London SE1 0EH
Information, advice, counselling. National helpline for families and friends of users.
Helpline: 0207 928 8898
www.adfam.org.uk

Families Anonymous
The Doddington and Rollo Community Association
Charlotte Despard Avenue
Battersea
London SW11 5HD
Advice and support groups for families and friends.
Helpline: 0845 1200 660
www.familiesanonymous.org

Release
388 Old Street
London EC1V 9LT
Telephone advice for legal emergencies and drug information and advice.
Telephone: 0207 729 5255
Emergency helpline (24-hour): 0207 749 4034
www.release.org.uk

National Drugs Helpline
Free information and advice and support around drug issues.
Helpline (24-hour): 0800 77 66 00

FRANK
Drugs advice for young people (Home Office).
Helpline: 0800 77 66 00
www.talktofrank.com

The Alliance – Methadone and Beyond
35 Cavendish Road
London N4 1RP
Advocacy services for drug users in treatment or seeking treatment.
Telephone: 0208 374 4395
www.m-alliance.org.uk

CHAPTER 16

Drugs and the law

Greg Poulter

For many years our society has struggled to establish a set of rules and regulations which will keep in balance three distinct aims.

1 To facilitate the effective therapeutic use of drugs.
2 A reduction in the harm the misuse of drugs can cause to both the individual and society.
3 To allow individuals a level of freedom of choice in their use of drugs, whether it be recreational or therapeutic.

Various pieces of legislation have been passed to establish this framework and the two prime sources are the Misuse of Drugs Act 1971 and the Medicines Act 1968. Due to a rapidly changing drug scene, each Statute has been amended and reinforced innumerable times by subsequent primary and subordinate legislation and their interpretation and effectiveness are subject to European and international law.

The resulting basic framework of law is reasonably straightforward and comprehensible. However, considerable complexities can arise when the law is applied; the devil certainly does reside in the detail.

The law needs to have certainty to be effective and individuals need to know what substances are subject to regulation, what those regulations allow them to do with the relevant substances and what are the penalties for breaking those controls.

The starting point in understanding the law in relation to drugs is to establish what substances are being regulated. It is helpful to view the law as being neatly divided into two distinct parts, the civil law and the criminal law, with each part possessing its own body of law, institutions and personnel and its own definitions of the substances being regulated. There are also radically different penalties for breaching the rules.

■ Civil law

In this area of law we are primarily considering the use of medicines. The inspiration for the Medicines Act (MA) was the protection of the public from defective or flawed medicines. It is not primarily aimed at combating the illegal possession or supply of 'street' drugs. However, there is an overlap. Some drugs which are not listed as Controlled Drugs under the MA are used as 'street' drugs for recreational purposes, for example ketamine. Anyone producing or selling ketamine could face criminal law sanction under the MA.

The MA and relevant European Community's pharmaceutical directives are in part enforced by the Medicines and Healthcare Products Regulatory Agency (MHRA), formerly the Medicines Control Agency. The agency regulates any product which is defined as a 'medicinal product' and oversees the production, licensing and distribution of such products.

It is, however, a complex matter to arrive at an accurate definition of a medicinal product. The Codified Pharmaceutical Directive 2001/83/EEC sets out the following definition.

> Any substance or combination of substances presented for treating or preventing disease in human beings or animals.
> Any substance or combination of substances which may be administered to human beings or animals with a view to making a diagnosis or to restoring, correcting or modifying physiological function in a human being or animal is likewise considered a medicinal product.

This is an exceptionally widely drawn definition and would, if taken at face value, include almost all material eaten, drunk or smoked. The regulatory body, the MHRA, is guided in determining if a substance is a medicinal product by a number of factors, including EC directives, case law, both domestic and European, and an 'assessment of all available evidence'.

A substance that is defined as a medicinal product must not be supplied in the United Kingdom unless it has a product licence or it is specifically exempt, although even then it will still require marketing authorisation. No such licence or authorisation would be granted unless the product meets a statutory standard of safety, quality and efficacy. It is a little surprising that no pressure group has yet thought to challenge the MHRA in the courts for breach of statutory duty in not categorising tobacco as a 'medicinal product' as if so challenged, it could not be sold without a product licence. Although tobacco could possibly meet quality and efficacy criteria, with 120 000 people a year dying prematurely, its safety might be questioned.

Once a substance is established as a medicinal product it is placed on one of three lists which are in part created by the MA.

- *Prescription-only medicines (POM)*. These can only be supplied under medical supervision and there is maximum control over their use and supply.
- *Pharmacy medicines*. If it is established that a medicine is safe for use with pharmacist supervision, then the medicine will be placed on this list.
- *The General Sales List*. Where it has been demonstrated that there is no need for professional advice or supervision in the use of the substance as a medicine, it can be placed on the General Sales List and there is minimal regulation over its supply.

■ Criminal law

The main piece of legislation in the criminal law is the Misuse of Drugs Act 1971 and the substances regulated by this statute are normally referred to as Controlled Drugs (CD). The Act conveniently contains a list of such drugs and these lists are referred to as Classes A, B and C. If a substance is placed into one of these classes it should be referred to as a Controlled Drug and where it is pharmaceutically produced, it should have 'CD' imprinted somewhere on its packaging.

The term 'illegal drug' is sometimes inaccurately used. A drug cannot in itself be illegal, whether it be cannabis, heroin, crack or temazepam, but what an individual might do with that substance can be illegal, i.e. they might possess, supply or produce it without authority. It is their actions that are illegal not the drug itself.

■ Misuse of Drugs Act (MDA)

This Act seeks to regulate the importation and exportation, production and possession of certain drugs that are considered 'dangerous or otherwise harmful'. The Act provides delegated powers to make regulations known as the Misuse of Drugs Regulations.

The MDA creates a number of criminal offences regarding the possession of Controlled Drugs. Thus Section 5(1) says:

> ... it shall not be lawful for a person to have a Controlled Drug in their *possession*.

Section 4(1) makes it an offence:

> to *supply* or *offer to supply* a Controlled Drug to another.

Section 5(3) makes it an offence:

> for a person to have a Controlled Drug in their possession, whether lawfully or not, with *intent to supply* it to another.

If the law stopped here then doctors and pharmacists could not undertake their work, as every time they provided their patient with dihydrocodeine or temazepam they would be committing an offence. Fortunately, the law provides a number of exceptions to the above offences, enabling doctors to prescribe and supply appropriate drugs in the course of their work.

■ What is a 'Controlled Drug'?

The MDA does not attempt to provide a definition of the dangerous drugs that it seeks to regulate. Rather, it sets out a series of lists of drugs which are described as 'Controlled Drugs'.

There are two groups of lists: the Classes and the Schedules.

Classes

The first group is found in Schedule 2 to the MDA and is referred to as the Classes. As might be expected, Controlled Drugs are not all treated the same under the law. There is a type of hierarchy of danger and those drugs which are viewed as the most dangerous and harmful and therefore attract the greatest penalty are placed in *Class A*. Diamorphine, cocaine and lysergide are examples of such drugs and the maximum penalty for unlawfully supplying one of these drugs is life imprisonment and/or an unlimited fine.

In *Class B* are the drugs which are viewed as less serious, such as amphetamine, codeine and methylamphetamine. The maximum penalty for unlawfully supplying a drug in this class is currently 14 years and/or an unlimited fine.

Class C contains the remaining Controlled Drugs, such as diazepam and temazepam, for which the current maximum penalty for supplying is five years and/or an unlimited fine.

In many cases any substance which is structurally derived from or is in any stereo-isometric form or salt of the substance named in the class is also controlled.

The sole function of the Classes is to set out the level of penalty for an offence associated with a particular Controlled Drug.

Schedules

The second group of lists is found in five Schedules contained in the Misuse of Drugs Regulations 1985 (as amended). The Schedules deal with far more complex areas of law than the Classes. The Schedule in which a particular Controlled Drug is placed dictates who can lawfully possess or supply it, how it must be stored, whether a GP can prescribe it, the form of the prescription, etc.

In Schedule 1 are drugs which are viewed as possessing no therapeutic value, so they cannot be prescribed. In this Schedule is lysergide. The remaining four Schedules impose different levels of control on the drugs contained within them. Those in Schedule 2 are subject to the most control with Schedule 5 the least. Schedule 2 drugs include dihydrocodeine, cocaine, diamorphine, methadone and pethidine. Schedule 3 includes chlorophentermine, mazindol and temazepam. Schedule 4 includes diazepam, lorazepam and nitrazepam.

Section 5 of the MDA makes it an offence to possess a Controlled Drug. However, under Regulation 10(1) of the Misuse of Drugs Regulations a practitioner or pharmacist may possess and supply a drug contained in Schedules 2–4. It is this regulation which gives authority to doctors to have a Controlled Drug in their possession and to administer it according to their clinical judgement. However, a specific licence is required before practitioners can prescribe cocaine, diamorphine or dipipanone to treat a dependency on those drugs, although any doctor can prescribe those drugs for other purposes. Any doctor may prescribe methadone for an opiate user.

As far as the patient is concerned, Regulation 10(2) protects them as follows.

> a person may have in his possession any drug specified in Schedule 2 or 3 for administration for medical, dental or veterinary purposes in accordance with the direction of a practitioner.

As a general rule Controlled Drugs contained in Schedules 2–4 can only be supplied by a practitioner or pharmacist and those in Schedules 2 and 3 can only be lawfully possessed by a member of the public if these drugs have been prescribed to them. Anyone can possess a Schedule 4 (ii) drug provided it is a medicinal product, i.e. in the form in which it is intended to be taken.

There are, of course, other categories of people who might possess or supply a Controlled Drug without committing an offence, providing they are doing so in the course of their profession or business, for example police officers, those engaged in the business of the Post Office or forensic examination in a laboratory, carriers, etc.

Any person may possess Schedule 5 drugs. These are various dilute, small-dose, non-injectable products that can often be sold without prescription by a pharmacist. They include cough medicines, antidiarrhoea agents and mild painkillers. Once bought, they cannot be supplied to someone else, an injunction that is rarely enforced.

Each Controlled Drug will have two listings, one in the Classes and one in the Schedules, so, for example, diamorphine is in Class A and Schedule 2 and amphetamine is in Class B and Schedule 2.

Certain drugs in Class B will be classified as Class A drugs if prepared for injecting.

The Act allows considerable flexibility to the Home Office to amend the Schedules and Classes. It is a relatively simple matter for new substances to be brought into control, as with anabolic steroids, which were introduced into Class C, Schedule 4. Existing Controlled Drugs can also be moved within the Schedules as with temazepam which, although it remains in Class C, was moved from Schedule 4 to Schedule 3. Thus it is now an offence to possess temazepam unless personally prescribed whereas formerly it was only an offence to supply it other than under a prescription. Flunitrazepam (Rohypnol) was moved up the Schedules to make possession an offence. The procedure that must be undertaken by the Home Office before such amendments can be made includes wide consultation, particularly with the Advisory Council on the Misuse of Drugs (ACMD).

■ Double scripting

If a patient obtains a prescription of Controlled Drugs from Dr A and then obtains a second prescription from Dr B without disclosing the first prescription, the patient will be in lawful possession of the drugs from Dr A but in unlawful possession of the drugs from Dr B.

■ Dishonestly obtaining Controlled Drugs

The Misuse of Drugs Regulations 10(2) provide that if a patient makes a declaration or statement to a prescribing doctor which 'was false in any (material) particular, for the purpose of obtaining the supply or prescription', the patient will be in unlawful possession of those prescribed drugs. Consequently if a patient misleads a doctor about the need for a particular drug, for example a patient lies about being dependent on heroin so as to obtain a methadone script, they are in unlawful possession of the methadone even though it has been prescribed to them by a practitioner.

■ Common offences

It is helpful for professionals working with individuals who are using street drugs to have a basic understanding of the more common offences.

The majority of people who come into contact with the criminal justice system are arrested for simple *possession* of a Controlled Drug. For the prosecution to establish this offence, it is necessary to show:

- that the substance was in the possession or control of the defendant
- that the substance was in fact a Controlled Drug
- that the defendant knew of the existence of the substance.

Many people arrested by the police in possession of a small quantity of a Controlled Drug will not be charged but will receive a 'caution', that is, a formal warning. For young people there is a reprimand and warning system followed on a third offence by the young person being charged with an offence of possession and being taken to court. For an adult, even if they are charged with the offence of possession and have to attend the court, the most likely sentence is a fine. It is now most unusual for an individual to receive a prison sentence for simple possession.

With regard to *supply* offences, there are a number of different categories. The two main ones are possession with intent to supply and actual supply. A wide range of activities involving Controlled Drugs can be classified as supplying and thus incur the possibility of a serious sentence. It is not necessary to show some benefit accruing to the supplier to make them guilty of the crime. If an individual simply gives or shares a Controlled Drug with another they commit the offence, so sharing a 'spliff' or 'joint' with a friend could be viewed as supplying cannabis. It would be an offence of 'possession with intent to supply' for a person to look after an ecstasy tablet for a friend. If two people club together to buy some cocaine, the person who goes to buy the drug would be committing a similar offence.

The consequences, on conviction, for the most minor of supply-type offences are frequently very serious. The 'entry point' for sentence is normally custodial. The supply of Class A drugs, even social supply of small amounts for no profit, will commonly attract a prison sentence of between 18 months and three years. Where there appears to be a profit motive, then 3–5-year sentences are very frequent. The fact that the defendant has no previous convictions may not substantially affect the sentence.

■ Street prices

The cost of street drugs to the user is a good indicator of availability. Shortages may push the prices up while gluts can cause the price to fall. However, it is a remarkable, if not disturbing feature of the street scene that prices are at least stable and in many situations, have fallen in recent years. In most parts of the United Kingdom 1/8th ounce of cannabis resin will currently sell for £10 and increasingly for as little as £5. Such an amount can produce up to 25 spliffs, depending on taste. Amphetamine costs between £5 and £10 per gram and ecstasy between £2 and £5 per tablet. The cost of heroin has been falling and a full gram will cost £30–50 in most parts of the United Kingdom. Heroin is also sold in individual bags and the weight of drug in these bags appears to be increasing. Cocaine can cost between £40 and £60 per gram. These drugs are also readily available in most parts of the United Kingdom.

■ Drug activities on premises

Section 8 of the MDA makes it an offence for an individual, who is the occupier or is concerned in the management of premises, to knowingly permit or suffer certain drug activities to take place. The activities in question are:

- the production or supply or offering to supply Controlled Drugs where such production or supply is unlawful
- the preparation of opium for smoking
- the smoking of cannabis, cannabis resin or prepared opium.

The use of other Controlled Drugs is not presently included in the section. The Home Office has considered extending the section to cover all Controlled Drugs but at present has postponed a decision.

This section imposes quite an onerous obligation on those affected by it. They must do all they reasonably can to stop the relevant activities taking place. If they fail in this responsibility then they can face serious sanctions which can result in imprisonment, as happened to two housing workers based in Cambridge who were prosecuted under this section.

■ Paraphernalia

Before August 2003 it was an offence under Section 9A of the MDA to knowingly supply any article that was to be used for the taking of a street drug. On the recommendation of many health professionals and the ACMD, the law was amended. From 1 August 2003 it is no longer an offence for doctors, pharmacists and drug workers to supply swabs, filters, sterile water, certain mixing utensils (e.g. spoons, bowls, cups and dishes) and citric acid to drug users who have obtained Controlled Drugs such as heroin and cocaine without a prescription.

■ Drugs and driving

There is an offence of driving a motor vehicle while unfit through drink or drugs. Most successful drink-driving convictions are based on the legal presumption that if the proportion of alcohol to breath is over a certain level then the driver is unfit and the offence is committed. No such provision is available for drug-driving matters. In these cases the prosecution must prove:

- that the driver was unfit, often based on the evidence of the medical examiner called by the police, and
- that the driver was unfit through drugs.

The law relating to driving while unfit applies equally to prescribed and non-prescribed drugs. It is not a defence to a charge of driving while unfit through drugs that the driver was unfit through a prescribed drug which had been taken in accordance with the doctor's directions.

For a number of years there has been grave concern on the part of many senior police officers that there are significant numbers of drivers who are unfit through drugs and there have been frequent calls for a radical overhaul of the law.

Prescribing practitioners do have responsibilities in this area. Guidelines are issued by the Driver and Vehicle Licensing Agency (DVLA) with regard to driving and drugs and these are obtainable from either the Stationery Office or the DVLA. It is possible that a prescribing practitioner could be viewed as negligent if he or she does not advise a patient as to the dangers of driving if the medication prescribed might affect their driving ability. With regard to prescribed methadone, the DVLA considers that a person should not be driving if they are in receipt of injectable methadone. If they receive the drug in any other form, then it is up to the doctor's clinical judgement as to whether the patient should continue to drive. Where a patient is driving and putting other road users at risk because they are impaired through their prescribed drugs, a doctor is quite entitled to notify the appropriate authorities, be it DVLA or the police.

■ Cannabis

In January 2004, the law on cannabis was amended. The possession and supply of cannabis remains a criminal offence; however, the drug is moved from Class B to Class C and the guidance to police officers, as to how they deal with the possession of the drug, has been amended.

The practical result of this is that the majority of adults who are found in possession of cannabis will not be arrested but will instead receive a written or verbal warning, which will be recorded at least at the local police station. This will form part of their criminal record and in certain circumstances may be disclosed on a criminal record check for employment and for other purposes. Subsequent offences of possession may result in a caution or a criminal conviction and a fine. If there is an aggravating element such as smoking in public or near a school or blowing smoke into a police officer's face, then this could result in the individual's immediate arrest and a resulting criminal conviction and record.

Young people aged 17 years or under will still immediately be arrested and dealt with under the youth cautioning procedures, which will result in a criminal record. If they commit a third offence they will go to the Youth Court and receive a criminal conviction.

It is still uncertain as to which Schedule cannabis might be moved and whether cannabis or any derivative of the plant will be capable of being prescribed. There is a substantial amount of research being undertaken and the government still needs to make a decision.

■ The role of the GP

The importance of GPs working in co-operation with local drug projects to deal effectively with drug dependency issues cannot be overemphasised. Many of these local agencies are able to provide guidance and support to GPs and their drug-dependent patients and, after an assessment of the patient, will make recommendations for prescribing. However, it is important that GPs do not delegate their clinical decisions to others. It remains the doctor's legal responsibility to ensure that an appropriate prescription is made.

It is no longer a requirement for a doctor who 'attends' a person suspected of addiction to specified drugs to notify the Chief Medical Officer at the Home Office as the 'Addicts Register' has been discontinued.

Key points

- The law in relation to drugs is a rapidly changing area and is never far from controversy.
- Health professionals should be aware of changes in the law and ensure that their working practices are lawful.
- Appropriate and lawful policies must be in place, kept under review and adhered to by all staff.
- Prescribing doctors must remember that the medicolegal responsibility for prescriptions they write rests with them.
- Advice to drug users about safe driving, whether or not they are in treatment, is important.

■ Useful contacts

Release
388 Old Street
London EC1V 9LT
Telephone advice for legal emergencies and drug information and advice.
Telephone: 0207 729 5255
Emergency helpline (24-hour): 0207 749 4034
www.release.org.uk

Driver and Vehicle Licensing Agency (DVLA)
Longview Road
Swansea SA6 7JL
Telephone: 01792 782341
www.dvla.gov.uk

CHAPTER 17

Training, continuing professional development and appraisal

Linda Harris

This chapter considers some of the ways in which generalist GPs can acquire skills and competencies in the field of substance misuse and how this can be positively presented in their appraisal. For the majority of GPs, learning and updating in drug misuse will form just one part of the many facets of their work and will be included within the overall portfolio of their continuing professional development (CPD). Annual appraisal is an opportunity to review this.

Appraisal for GPs

Annual appraisal for GPs was introduced in 2002 and is co-ordinated by primary care trusts (PCTs), who have the ultimate responsibility for ensuring appraisal is provided in accordance with standards defined by the General Practitioners' Committee (GPC) and the RCGP. Running parallel to this process is revalidation. This applies to all doctors and will be implemented by the General Medical Council (GMC) from 2005. Revalidation combines traditional registration with a licence to practise, which is revalidated every five years. Appraisal is not revalidation nor is it assessment.

- *Revalidation* aims to ensure that GPs are working to acceptable minimum standards of fitness to practice.
- *Assessment* may, in part, inform appraisal but its role is to test performance against a set of criteria.
- *Appraisal* is a positive review process that is educational, formative and confidential. It enables GPs to reflect on all aspects of their work with a colleague, obtain feedback on their past performance and identify development needs.

GPs are advised to utilise the annual appraisal process and associated documentation to meet the requirements for GMC revalidation against the seven headings of *Good Medical Practice*. See the following websites:
www.gmc-uk.org/revalidation
www.doh.gov.uk/gpappraisal

■ Personal development planning for GPs wishing to further their knowledge in drug misuse

Appraisal is an opportunity to reflect on one's personal and development needs. A personal development plan (PDP) is a useful tool to help individuals plan to meet those needs. It can be used as a basis for deciding what to address during the next year. The PDP should include personal development objectives in the management of drug misuse in primary care and a range of development activities designed to help achieve them. Generalists will need to take account of their professional needs, the requirements of the practice and their personal ambitions.

Key stages in preparing a plan are:

- identifying current level of competence
- specifying competencies to develop
- deciding how to develop these competencies and by when
- setting performance criteria to be achieved as a result of the development
- taking development action
- deciding how and when to review progress.

The Update Personal Development Plan is simple, well-structured and easy to use; template available at www.doctorupdate.net.

As with all areas of practice, the process of CPD in substance misuse should:

- be purposeful and personally motivating
- raise individual awareness
- consider the development needs of the practice
- be evidence based where possible
- develop knowledge of and opportunities for research and development
- place the individual at the centre of the educational process.

■ Learning styles

Generally speaking, we learn on our own, in our own particular individual way. Learning depends on many factors, many of them personal. If you explore your preferred learning modalities you will become a better learner. For help with this, go to the following website and search for 'learning': www.hcc.hawaii.edu/search.html

■ What are the skills and competencies needed for GPs working with substance misusers?

The RCGP, in conjunction with *Skills for Health* (Drug and Alcohol National Occupational Standards) and Substance Misuse Management in General

Practice (SMMGP), has developed a set of competencies for GPs who wish to provide services for drug users as a National Enhanced Service (NES) under the new Contract. The competencies have been mapped across to learning outcomes which can then be used by GPs planning their personal development. These competencies form the basis of the learning outcomes for the RCGP Part 1 Certificate course in the management of drug misuse for which this book is part of the recommended reading.

■ RCGP national drug misuse training programme

This programme was established in January 2001 and is funded by the Department of Health. It is responsible for the Part 1 Certificate course, due to be launched in June 2004, which is a useful way of acquiring the skills and competencies needed for generalist GPs providing a LES/NES. In addition to local face-to-face delivery, the course uses modern distance learning methodology and includes online access to lectures and presentations, self-assessment questionnaires and discussion groups for support and peer group learning. It will become multidisciplinary, but is only GPs in the first year. Clinicians with an appropriate level of experience or who have successfully completed Part 1 can go on to take Part 2 of the Certificate, which has been available since September 2001. If completed successfully and he/she continues to have CPD and appraisal in this specialist area, this will accredit a GP to work as a GP with a special interest in drug misuse (GPwSI).

■ RCGP regional leads in substance misuse

The RCGP national drug misuse training programme has appointed a number of GPs with expertise in drug misuse to provide support and information to local clinical leads and commissioners of primary care substance misuse services. They also have skills in education and training. The regional leads host clinical networks and regional training events to share best practice and offer peer support to GPs working with drug users. They will act as advisers and appraisers for GPwSIs in their region. They provide an important strategic link between local clinicians, the RCGP and the National Treatment Agency regional managers.

■ Action learning

One of the strengths of the RCGP courses in substance misuse is their use of mentoring and action learning in order to create productive and vibrant learning environments. The principle of action learning is to bring together a small number of practitioners, ideally from neighbouring localities, to discuss and share their understanding of a topic area or a piece of project work.

There are a number of factors that contribute to successful action learning.

- Meet in protected learning time and preferably at a neutral meeting place to minimise interruptions.
- Identify learning outcomes for the meeting beforehand and share them with the whole group, including any preparatory reading or external activities such as field visits or online learning.
- Share examples of best practice with other members of the group.
- Draw on the resources within the group to solve problems, find answers to questions or constructively criticise the evidence base to enhance understanding of a subject area.

Positive feedback from GPs who complete elements of their CPD through action learning includes:

- added value of working with one's peers and having access to a wider network of practitioners
- the usefulness of rapid access to expertise from within the group
- support and coaching from an experienced mentor
- the benefits of group working over professional isolation
- opportunities for feedback regarding professional and clinical practice from within the group.

■ Keeping a personal learning portfolio

Far from being yet another administrative task to burden GPs whose desks are already heaving with paper, putting together a portfolio of learning can be embraced within ordinary day-to-day work. It is used not only as a record of activities but as a tool to plan your learning.

The easiest way of keeping a portfolio is to file all educational activities and learning opportunities in chronological order throughout the annual appraisal cycle. This will ensure you keep your records up to date but a thematic approach to organising your portfolio will provide your appraiser and yourself with a better indication of how your learning activities are addressing specific learning needs and objectives.

■ Example of a themed approach to maintaining evidence of learning in substance misuse

Clinical practice
- Attendance at lectures and workshops on clinical management of substance misuse.
- Prescribing and therapeutics including the reading and understanding of local and national protocols in substance misuse.
- Field visits to other services.
- Clinical attachments with addiction specialists.
- Clinical skills workshops in motivational interviewing.

Learning from a clinical network

This method is increasing in popularity since the advent of email and is reliant on a cohort of individuals committed to sharing best practice and who see the value of drawing on the experience and advice of peers accessible through the Internet medium. One way of introducing yourself to a network is through an organised website such as the SMMGP website (*see* Useful contacts list).

Clinical networks can be local, regional or national and offer a flexible and convenient way to seek answers to queries and share experience and best practice. The SMMGP website not only has a wealth of materials and resources to tap into, including up-to-date information on the RCGP Certificate courses, but also hosts discussion forums and an 'online surgery' where questions on the management of substance misuse can be posted up and answers sought from the whole network.

National policy initiatives

- Policy documents such as government consultation documents and Green and White Papers will keep you abreast of political drivers in the drug misuse field.
- The website for the National Drug Strategy, a joint project of the Home Office and the Department of Health, is a useful resource (www.drugs.gov.uk).
- The National Treatment Agency website contains a wealth of information including the NTA corporate strategy, hyperlinks to national guidelines, information on service standards including drug and alcohol national occupational standards, and National Service Framework (*Models of Care*) information (www.nta.nhs.uk).

Learning from critical incidents and complaints

As a GP you will be keeping a record of untoward incidents and it is important to review the procedures in place if something doesn't go well so that the right lessons can be learnt. Ask the following questions when something goes wrong in the care of a drug user.

- What happened?
- How did it affect the patient, you, the practice?
- Why did it happen?
- What steps can be taken to avoid similar events in future?
- What learning needs are revealed by the event?
- How will these needs be met?

Audit and other written projects

Regular audits will be a requirement for GPs providing an NES for drug users. Suggested topics are:

- audit of prescribing and adherence to guidelines in prescribing practice
- hepatitis B screening and immunisation rates.

Using a reflective log book

Choose a couple of patients with drug use problems whom you are looking after and write a narrative on their progress. Alternatively, look at a couple of randomly selected patients. Training practices may have access to audio and video material to review consultation and intervention skills.

Key points

- Substance misuse is just one small part of the knowledge base required of general practitioners.
- There is a wide range and choice of resources and learning opportunities around substance misuse.
- Maintaining and developing knowledge and skills requires CPD in substance misuse that is reviewed through the appraisal process.

■ Useful contacts

RCGP national drug misuse training programme
Frazer House
32–38 Leman Street
London E1 8EW
Telephone: 0207 173 6092
Email: mmurnane@rcgp.org.uk
www.smmgp.co.uk/html/rcgp.htm

Substance Misuse Management in General Practice (SMMGP)
This is a network to support GPs and other members of the primary healthcare team who work with substance misuse. The project team produces the Substance Misuse Management in General Practice newsletter (*Network*) and, in collaboration with the RCGP, organises the annual RCGP conference Managing Drug Users in General Practice.
www.smmgp.co.uk

■ Summary of useful websites

www.gmc-uk.org/revalidation
www.doh.gov.uk/gpappraisal
www.doctorupdate.net
www.hcc.hawaii.edu/search.html
www.smmgp.co.uk
www.drugs.gov.uk
www.nta.nhs.uk

Index